Carl Jung and the Evolutionary Sciences

I0092181

This book revaluates Carl Jung's ideas in the context of contemporary research in the evolutionary sciences. Recent work in developmental biology, as well as experimental and psychedelic neuroscience, has provided empirical evidence that supports some of Jung's central claims about the nature and evolution of consciousness. Beginning with a historical contextualisation of the genesis of Jung's evolutionary thought and its roots in the work of the nineteenth-century *Naturphilosophen*, the book then outlines a model of analytical psychology grounded in modern theories of brain development and life history theory. The book also explores research on evolved sex-based differences and their relevance to Jung's concept of the anima and animus.

Seeking to build bridges between analytical psychology and contemporary evolutionary studies and associated fields, this book will appeal to scholars of analytical and depth psychology, as well as researchers in the evolutionary and brain sciences.

Gary Clark is currently a Visiting Research Fellow in the School of Medical Sciences at the University of Adelaide in Australia. Since 2012, he has been a member of School's Biological Anthropology and Comparative Anatomy Unit. His research focus includes the evolution of music, palaeoanthropology and evolutionary approaches to analytical psychology.

'Clark strengthens the biological view of analytical psychology with this outstanding, scholarly, and rigorous exploration. Integrating neuroscience, contemporary evolutionary theory, anthropology, and many other disciplines, he shows how a conceptually precise and balanced multi-disciplinary analysis can inform and enlighten analytical psychology. Overall a fantastic addition to the growing body of scholarship that blends clinical insight with empirical research and critical social science insights.'

Erik Goodwyn, MD, Co-editor-in-chief, *International Journal of Jungian Studies,* author of *The Neurobiology of the Gods* (Routledge, 2012).

'Brimming with rich, well researched and widely applied socio-anthropological insights, Dr Clark's important contribution infuses the reader with renewed enthusiasm to explore depth psychology within the context of neuroscientific findings.'

Dr Elizabeth Brodersen, Jungian Training analyst and Supervisor, CGJIZ and editor of *Jungian Dimensions of the Mourning Process, Burial Rituals and Access to the Land of the Dead; Intimations of Immortality* (Routledge, 2024).

'It is difficult to overstate the range and depth of Gary Clark's erudition. Rooting himself in the tradition of *Naturphilosophie*, he weaves perspectives from evolutionary theory, primatology, psychology, comparative religion, anthropology and philosophy in a compelling synthesis, arguing that much contemporary post-Jungian theory represents an abandonment, indeed, a betrayal of Jung's original project and vision for the study of the collective unconscious. In the process, he gives new meaning and relevance to Jung's concepts of anima and animus, eros and logos and much else besides. An inspired and inspiring *tour de force*.'

Daniel Burston, author of *Anti-Semitism and Analytical Psychology: Jung, Politics and Culture* (Routledge, 2021).

COMPARATIVE PSYCHOANALYSIS BOOK SERIES
DAVID HENDERSON & JON MILLS
Series Editors

Comparative Psychoanalysis studies controversy and dialogue in psychoanalysis. Intellectual, personal, and institutional conflict are endemic to the history of psychoanalysis. Alongside this there are creative efforts to establish understanding and communication among differing perspectives. Comparative methodologies are encouraged among all schools of psychoanalysis regardless of topic, theoretical or clinical orientation, or application to the behavioral sciences and humanities including historical reassessments, conceptual clarification, clinical exploration, reflections on the future of applied psychoanalytic thought, and attempts to articulate the conditions for fruitful dialogue. All subject matters in the arts and humanities, philosophy, anthropology, cultural studies, and the human sciences are ripe for comparative investigation within the frameworks of theoretical, clinical, and applied psychoanalysis. As an inherently interdisciplinary field of study, psychoanalysis requires a robust understanding of comparative methodology. Controversial discussions and criticism are invited. In the spirit of pluralism, Comparative Psychoanalysis is open to any theoretical school in the history of the psychoanalytic movement that offers novel critique, integration, and important insights in comparative scholarship.

Titles in this series:

The Psychoanalytic Understanding of Consciousness, Free Will, Language, and Reason: What Makes Us Human? *By Robert Samuels*

Carl Jung and the Evolutionary Sciences: A New Vision for Analytical Psychology *By Gary Clark*

Carl Jung and the Evolutionary Sciences

A New Vision for Analytical Psychology

Gary Clark

Routledge
Taylor & Francis Group

LONDON AND NEW YORK

Designed cover image: Ernst Haeckel's Hummingbirds,
from *Art Forms in Nature*, 1904.

First published 2025
by Routledge
4 Park Square, Milton Park, Abingdon, Oxon OX14 4RN

and by Routledge
605 Third Avenue, New York, NY 10158

*Routledge is an imprint of the Taylor & Francis Group, an
informa business*

British Library Cataloguing-in-Publication Data
A catalogue record for this book is available from the
British Library

ISBN: 978-1-032-62453-2 (hbk)
ISBN: 978-1-032-62451-8 (pbk)
ISBN: 978-1-032-62454-9 (ebk)

DOI: 10.4324/9781032624549

Typeset in Times New Roman
by KnowledgeWorks Global Ltd.

Contents

Introduction

Carl Jung was fully aware that he was mapping unexplored psychological terrain in his investigations into the deep unconscious layers of the mind. Jung commented on pioneers who follow a path that is incommensurate with that of their contemporaries, noting the 'dangers' and 'loneliness' such an undertaking may entail. Even though he is speaking in the third person, these reflections no doubt refer to his own trajectory of intellectual enquiry: 'there are things that are not yet true today, perhaps we dare not find them true, but tomorrow they may be' (Jung 1992: 119). One of the main claims of this book is that Jung's 'tomorrow' has in many senses arrived and that advances in evolutionary and experimental neuroscience have vindicated many of his claims about the human psyche.

Throughout most of the twentieth century, Jung's ideas were on the whole rejected by the academic and scientific establishment – as his comment intimates. One of the few disciplines in which his ideas took hold was literary studies (Bodkin 1958; Singer 1986; Edinger 1986, 1990; Kimball 1997; Rowland 1999). Literature is one of the domains of culture where archetypal aspects of our species evolved neurobiology are most cogently expressed. Although Jung was an evolutionary empiricist, he was also an acutely sensitive reader of literature and poetry (Jung 1991: 67–134). In this sense, there was a natural fit between Jung's ideas and literary criticism. However, this is the exception that proved the rule. Throughout most of the twentieth century, serious academic consideration of Jung's thought among scientists, evolutionary theorists and anthropologists was rare.

As the twentieth century came to a close and we entered the twenty-first century, attitudes towards Jung began to shift. In 1990, Anthony Stevens published his ground-breaking evolutionary exploration of Jung's ideas *Archetype: A Natural History of the Self* which was consequently updated and reissued (Stevens 1990, 2002). E.O. Wilson, founder of the field of sociobiology and one of the most influential evolutionary theorists of the twentieth century, adopted an archetypal approach to cultural analysis in his 1999 *Consilience: The Unity of Knowledge* (Wilson 1999: 85 and 238). In 2008, Thomas Lawson

DOI: 10.4324/9781032624549-1

published his *Carl Jung, Darwin of the Mind* in which he defended Jung's evolutionary thought:

> Jung's theory propounds that a collective unconscious, structured by archetypes, evolved through natural selection, just as did the instincts. It postulates, further, that from this inherited unconscious, present in all humans, consciousness arose. The subsequent and, at least within the last six thousand years, rapid, evolution of consciousness can be charted in developments in civilizations through history.
>
> (Lawson 2008: 4)

In 2011, John Haule released his two-volume *Jung in the 21st Century*, a work that drew on what at the time were the most recent findings in neuroscience and brain evolution (Haule 2011a, 2011b). However, probably the most significant scientific development in recent years that provides support for Jungian ideas is the neuroimaging undertaken by researchers in psychedelic neuroscience. One of the pioneers of this field is Professor Robin Carhart-Harris who is currently the Director of the Neuroscape Psychedelics Division in the Department of Neurology at the University of California. Carhart-Harris has argued that psychedelics enable researchers to explore the unconscious dimensions of the mind in experimental and laboratory settings. Such exploration has been difficult in the past as the unconscious, being generally inaccessible to consciousness, is notoriously difficult to study in an empirical manner.

Psychedelics are renowned for their ability to dissolve the structures of ego consciousness and to bring unconscious content into awareness. Commenting on the underappreciated depths of the human mind in mainstream psychology and psychiatry, Carhart-Harris argues that the greatest value of psychedelics to modern research may be 'as a remedy for ignorance of the unconscious mind' (Carhart-Harris et al. 2014: 18). Significantly, Carhart-Harris endorses a Jungian approach to the content that surfaces in the acute psychedelic state, arguing that subjects often report experiencing archetypal material similar to the religious iconography studied by Jung.

Carhart-Harris argues that the psychedelic state may represent a phase transition from recently evolved secondary process brain systems associated with ego consciousness to phylogenetically ancient primary process systems (Carhart-Harris and Friston 2010; Carhart-Harris et al. 2014: 14). Using fMRI technology, Carhart-Harris and colleagues have been able to analyse changes in neural architecture and brain connectivity in subjects who have been administered psychedelic compounds. These neurological changes correlate with self-reports of ego dissolution and archetypal religious or mystical experiences that have profound cathartic and therapeutic value.

I have applied this model in my own formulation of an evolutionary conception of analytical psychology informed by psychedelic neuroscience (Clark 2020b, 2021, 2022). Correlations between archetypal religious experiences and neurobiological substrates suggest that such subjective experiences and their neural correlates are aspects of the same underlying phenomenon. This enables research-ers to develop a neurophenomenological conception of analytical psychology that avoids the pitfalls of dualism and reductive materialism, while also acknowledg-ing that the richness and subtlety of inner experience are nevertheless mediated by underlying neurobiological and neurochemical processes (Clark 2022). In my analysis of this research and its relevance to evolutionary conceptions of analytical psychology, I argued that a phase transition from higher cortical regions associated with ego consciousness to primary process brain systems characterises dreamlife, ritual and the human desire to alter consciousness. These phenomena seem to be unique to our species and have not been observed in any other primate species known to us. Consequently, I have argued that *Homo sapiens* is the Dionysian Primate (Clark 2022). This approach to analytical psychology will be central to the model outlined in this book.

Support for Jung's theories has also come from Jaak Panksepp, one of the major figures in neuroscience in the last half-century. Panksepp founded the discipline of affective neuroscience and was a pioneer in the study of homologous brain systems humans share with other mammals. He outlined this research in his seminal 1998 *Affective Neuroscience: The Foundations of Human and Animal Emotions*. In an article Panksepp wrote in 2017, just prior to his passing, with Antonio Alcaro and Stefano Carta entitled 'The Affective Core of the Self: A Neuro-Archetypical Per-spective on the Foundations of Human (and Animal) Subjectivity,' he connected Jung's ideas to contemporary neuroscience. For example, when noting Jung's be-lief that archetypes may be related to evolutionarily ancient subcortical brain sys-tems, Panksepp and colleagues write that 'such assertions by Jung were not only quite farsighted, but they actually open ways to connect his theory of the psyche with the most advanced scientific theories and discoveries of our day' (Alcaro, Carta, and Panksepp 2017).

Panksepp has developed the notion of homologous brain systems to explain affinities between the human brain and those of other mammals. In biology, the concept of homology describes the same trait in a number of different and often distantly related species. The most parsimonious explanation for homologous traits is that each species inherited the trait from a common ancestor. An example of ho-mology is the neurochemical oxytocin which in all mammals serves to bond moth-ers and infants. For example, human mothers share this system with elephants and mice. This is most likely due to the fact that oxytocin facilitated infant attachment in the very first mammals some 200 million years ago. It has remained a fundamen-tal aspect of all mammalian species ever since. In humans, it not only underpins attachment between mothers and infants but also seems to have been repurposed in social and sexual psychology, as well as in forms of social bonding involving music, ritual and dance (Dissanayake 2021). Oxytocin has come to be known as the love hormone (Carter 2022).

Jung never used the term homology. However, his concept of archetypes essen-tially describes the same phenomenon. Significantly, the concept of homology was developed by the English palaeontologist Richard Owen (1804–1892) in works such as *On the Archetype and Homologies of the Vertebrate Skeleton* (1848). This concept was to have an impact on Darwin who sought to explain homologous structures, much in the same way modern biologists do, as a result of inheritance from a common ancestor (Hall 1993: 58). Importantly, Owen developed the concept of homology through his study of the *Naturphilosophen*, a group of German philosophers and comparative anatomists who argued that the different animal species on earth share underlying anatomical archetypes, and that these archetypes differentiate to different degrees resulting in the different species on earth. Significantly, it is this German tradition in comparative anatomy that Jung's evolutionary ideas developed out of (Clark 2023). In Chapter 1, I explore the crucial role this tradition played in the genesis of Jung's evolutionary conception of the psyche.

One of the important influences on my own thinking is Chris Knight's 1995 book *Blood Relations: Menstruation and the Origins of Culture*. My evolutionary approach to analytical psychology is deeply indebted to Knight's theories and their elaboration by various other scholars (Knight 1988, 1995; Power, Sommer, and Watts 2013; Finnegan 2013; Knight and Lewis 2016). Particularly important in this context is the 2017 collection of essays *Human Origins: Contributions from Social Anthropology* (Power, Finnegan, and Callan 2017). Knight's book and this collection of essays provide a rich source of material that can assist in grounding analytical psychology in evolutionary anthropology. The connections between Knight's model and Jungian thought have yet to be explored in any great detail. I previously made a tentative effort to use Knight's model in a Jungian context (Clark 2020a).

Throughout this book, I build on that earlier essay through a more extensive exploration of the connections between Knight's theories and analytical psychology. This involves a discussion of blood symbolism, menstruation and female sociality in the work of a number of Jungians. For example, in her classic *Woman's Mysteries: Ancient and Modern*, Esther Harding explored from a Jungian perspective issues that Knight and colleagues approach from an evolutionary point of view. Erich Neumann in *The Fear of the Feminine* and Sylvia Perera in her *Descent to the Goddess: A Way of Initiation for Women* also focus on these issues from a Jungian perspective (Harding 1936; Perera 1981; Neumann 1994).

What these Jungian works share with Knight's model are certain assumptions about the role of female coalitions and symbolism in the human past. Much of this material focusses on the role of female reproductive cycles and sexuality, and the ways in which societies are structured around them. Where Knight's model is unique is that he offers a Darwinian explanation of these cultural phenomena, something Jungians have not really developed. In essence, Knight and colleagues argue that at some time in the evolutionary past, women began to create coalitions and forms of resistance against male dominance. By periodically withholding sex, and only agreeing to it once men had gone out hunting and brought back game to share with the community, women were effectively able to control male sexual and hunting behaviour. The consequences of this are that male reproductive effort was channelled into socially productive avenues that contributed to group cohesion.

This control of male sexual psychology and hunting behaviour laid the foundations of what we know of as egalitarianism. In terms of Darwinian selection, men who were more willing to respect female solidarity and share the bounty of the hunt with their partners, offspring and the broader community would have an evolutionary advantage over males who were less community minded. For example, if coalitions of women began preferring such generous mates and were also able to deter more socially aggressive and selfish males, such coalitions would effectively change the evolutionary trajectory of male psychology and social behaviour.

This model explains some of the most salient cross-cultural features in the ethnographic record, that is the association of female menstrual blood and the blood of animals. Both of these forms of blood are considered sacred and taboo. Such a sense of the sacredness of blood effectively creates boundaries that curtail male behaviour. Significantly, the sacredness of blood was one of the core features of Emile Durkheim's theory of the origins of religion outlined in his 1912 classic *The Elementary Forms of Religious Life*. It was also a theme that Jung developed in significant detail in his analysis of ritual and blood symbolism.

Jungian scholars have noted similarities between the work of Durkheim and Jung (Staude 1976; Greenwood 2013; Goodwyn 2014). However, they have not explored one of the prime reasons for those similarities – namely both Durkheim and Jung used the works of Baldwin Spencer (1860–1929) and Francis Gillen (1855–1912) in their writing on ritual, totemism and blood symbolism. In the late nineteenth and early twentieth centuries, Spencer and Gillen undertook research among the Aranda people, an Indigenous language group in Central Australia who live in the region surrounding the remote town of Alice Springs. Spencer and Gillen's *The Native Tribes of Central Australia* (1899) and *The Northern Tribes of Central Australia* (1904) had a profound impact on the nascent discipline of anthropology. Their works were revolutionary at the time so much so that they changed the trajectory of European intellectual history. Not only were their works key source texts for Jung and Durkheim, they were also used by Freud and Sir James Frazer among many others too numerous to mention (Morphy 1988, 1997).

One of the overarching themes of this book is the importance of Spencer and Gillen's research in the genesis of Jung's thought. However, like Durkheim, Jung did not develop an explicit evolutionary account of how blood actually became scared at some time during human evolution. Jung hints at its significance, and like Durkheim seems to be aware of its important role in terms of kinship and social structure. However, he provides no Darwinian explanation of how and why blood acquired its sacred status. Nor do other Jungians like Harding, Neumann and Perera.

In Chapter 2, I explore these issues in detail in terms of the early influences on Jung's thought. In Chapter 3, I explore them from the point of view of contemporary evolutionary theory and how research on sex-based differences may help illuminate the Jungian concepts of Eros and Logos. The concept of Eros has been used by Jungians to explore female symbolism in various cultural periods, which is often juxtaposed with Logos or the masculine principle. In my analysis,

I seek to connect this tradition in Jungian thought to Knight's evolutionary model. I also look at critiques of this aspect of Jungian thought from postmodern, poststructuralist and feminist perspectives. While such critiques highlight potential problems in Jung's analysis of sex-based differences and the polarity of Eros and Logos, I conclude that Jung's thought is basically correct and is supported by research in multiple disciplines, from anthropology to experimental psychology.

In Chapter 4, I deepen the analysis by critiquing Jung's views of fossil hominins such as *Homo erectus* and Neanderthals. The chapter outlines modern research in life history theory and brain ontogeny. These approaches show surprising affinities with Jung's thinking on the relationship between ontogeny and phylogeny. More specifically, the extension of human ontogeny to include an adolescent period of socio-cognitive development is one of the main traits that distinguishes humans from other primates. I explore these theories in order to update Jung's evolutionary model of consciousness emerging from a prior state of unconsciousness in both ontogeny and phylogeny. This chapter outlines the main theoretical component of the book regarding human brain evolution. That model is then explored further in Chapters 5 and 6 where I apply it to archaeological and ethnographic data.

Nietzsche famously wrote that philosophy tends to be 'a confession of faith on the part of its author, and a type of involuntary and unself-conscious memoir' (Nietzsche 2002: 8). That is definitely the case for this book. One of the prime motivations behind my research has been to make sense of certain experiences that have occurred within my own life.

My first degree was in classical music performance. Practising for exams involves intense concentration and discipline often for up to eight to ten hours a day. That focus seems to change how consciousness operates and on rare occasions a player may be rewarded with quite intense alterations of consciousness or what are sometimes called flow states. On one particular occasion during an exam about half-way through the recital, my sense of space and time became profoundly altered. The recital was in a large Gothic-style hall with very high rafters in which birds had built their nests. I had not noticed them before, but during the recital, the birds and their soft gentle song moved into the foreground of my awareness. On this occasion, my consciousness seemed to expand and fill the entire hall. More specifically, it entered the souls of the birds and *entered their song*. Of course, this sounds all but impossible from a rational perspective. How can the consciousness of a human being be *in* the song of a bird? However, being *in* or coextensive with the song and souls of these little birds is the best way to describe the *phenomenology* of the experience. My own body, the music I was playing, the souls of the birds and their song were of the same substance. That is they were consubstantial. There was also no sense of time – it could have been ten seconds or ten hours. There was no sense of individualised essences or beings. Space and time had fallen away and in their place was a state of transcendent euphoria. Afterwards, I was not quite sure what had happened. I retained a sense of deep well-being for about an hour after the concert.

This experience always stayed with me and I suspect it was one of the reasons why I took an interest in Jung as a student, often reading his works while neglecting my course work. I recognised those moments in the Gothic hall as the kind of experience Jung often referred to as *numinous*. As I went on to do other things, the experience melded into the background of my awareness and I tended to forget about it. I only began seriously contemplating its significance in recent years. The catalyst for that reawakened interest came from reading *Deciphering Ancient Minds: The Mystery of San Bushman Rock Art* by David Lewis-Williams and Sam Challis (Lewis-Williams and Challis 2011). What captured my interest was reading about how when shamans enter trance states, they will often speak of becoming a bird or another specific animal. On a rational level, such a statement makes little sense. But it describes with the utmost accuracy the experience I had during my recital. After reading *Deciphering Ancient Minds*, I began exploring these issues in much greater depth. The present book is the result of those investigations.

Another important personal factor influencing the ideas developed in this book is work I did with remote Indigenous people in the Central Deserts of Australia. In the early 2000s, I was completing a doctorate in literature and ecology with a focus on how Indigenous conceptions of the sacred influenced Anglo-Celtic poets and their writing about the Australian landscape. This involved reading quite a bit of anthropology. While I was finishing the thesis, I decided to spend some time teaching in Central Australia – and as opposed to merely reading about Indigenous culture, I decided I would live with the people and experience their culture firsthand. I ended up teaching for several years developing not only a unique insight into traditional culture, but also forming some very precious friendships.

During my time living in Central Australia, I hunted kangaroos, gathered bush tucker and participated in ceremonial activity. A lot of this time was spent with older members of the community who had not seen white people until their teenage years in the 1950s and 1960s. Those old people are the last generation to have memories of pre-contact times. These were important experiences; I was given the opportunity to drink kangaroo blood from a freshly cooked carcass (the prerogative of males only) and was invited to participate in sacred ceremonial activity. The chapters in this book that deal with Indigenous ritual and symbolism essentially grew out of those very personal experiences. Those experiences have stayed with me over the years and much of my research has been directed at deepening my understanding of these aspects of Indigenous spiritual life. I will always remain grateful to the people who welcomed me into their community and shared their culture with me.

One particular incident always stays with me. One day, an Aboriginal colleague placed his arm on my shoulder and said: 'You see that hill. I'm that one. That one honey ant man. He come all the way from Papunya.' The man had very limited English and had grown up in the remote desert regions with minimal contact with the broader Australian community. He lived in a community about 400 kilometres from Papunya, another remote desert settlement. In that short phrase, he was recounting the travels of ancestral beings during the Dreaming over vast stretches of country – travels that are immortalised in the Songlines that traverse the continent of Australia.

For him, the honey ant ancestor, the physical embodiment of that ancestor in features of the landscape, the actual honey ants that are an important food source in the desert, as well as his own being were in his view of the same substance; as he said: 'I'm that one.' Essentially his totem was the honey ant. This means his spirit was vivified in his mother's womb by the honey ant ancestor whose body transformed into the hill during the Dreaming or creative period. Additionally, during ritual and dreamlife, he maintains contact with that ancestral being. Significantly, the concept of the Dreaming (*alcheringa* in Aranda) was an important aspect of Jung's understanding of ritual and social organisation that he derived from his reading of Spencer and Gillen. This connection will be explored in Chapter 2.

As I was doing research for this book, I began to realise the important role Spencer and Gillen played in the genesis of Jung's thought. It also became clear that this influence had tended to be overlooked in Jungian scholarship and that my experiences gave me unique insight into the sources of Jung's writings on anthropology. When I was teaching in Central Australia, we would often drive to Alice Springs on weekends for a drink at the local pub. These drives were often up to eight or nine hours as the communities I was living in were deep in the remote desert regions. Alice Springs is a remote and quite small town. However, it serves as the administrative hub for the remote Indigenous communities not only in the surrounding McDonnel Ranges but also deeper into the remote desert regions. Despite its small size compared to other Australian towns, it is the only major regional administrative centre in the vast regions of the Australia's Central deserts.

Importantly, it is in Alice Springs that Spencer and Gillen did their field work over a century ago. For years, I had spent time in Alice and was fascinated by its history and had written numerous articles on cultural exchange and anthropology in the region. In terms of the trajectory of nineteenth- and early twentieth-century European intellectual history, Alice Springs was pivotal. Importantly, the German Missionary Carl Strehlow, who ran the Lutheran Mission at Hermannsburg a few hours' drive from Alice, was also an important figure of the period – although he is less known than Spencer and Gillen, with his works only ever being published in German. His influential work on myth and linguistics, *Die Aranda- und Loritja-Stämme in Zentral-Australien* (1907–1920), became one of the central texts in the emerging discipline of anthropology. Marcel Mauss wrote positive reviews of the work for Durkheim's journal *L'Année sociologique* (Mauss 1910, 1913). In his discussion, Mauss evocatively compared Strehlow's work to ancient Hindu hymns and chants, remarking that the volumes represented a form of an Aranda Rig Veda (Kenny 2013: 242).

Having been familiar with the work of Strehlow and Spencer and Gillen for years and having lived in the region where they did their field work, I realised I had a unique perspective on important influences upon Jung's thought that scholars from Europe or America lacked. This was obviously an accident of geography – I happen to live where the research was undertaken that had such a profound impact on the nascent discipline of anthropology and the development of psychoanalysis and analytical psychology.

It was these personal factors that resulted in this book having an Australian focus. The majority of the anthropological material I discuss is Australian. But this is not only because that material is an intrinsic part of my background – the emphasis results from the fact that Australian ethnography had a significant impact on the genesis of Jung's thought. However, it has not to my knowledge been explored in any detail. In focussing on this dimension of Jung's thought, I was able to both deepen my knowledge of material I was already familiar with as well as fill lacunae in the extant analytical psychology literature.

In this study, I also draw on my own research in palaeoanthropology. For a number of years, I have been a Research Fellow in the Biological Anthropology and Comparative Anatomy Unit in the Medical School at The University of Adelaide. Our research has focussed on the early stages of human evolution going back to the early Pliocene some four and a half millions years ago. We have published papers on the fossil species *Ardipithecus ramidus* as well as *Homo erectus* and early Australian fossils (Clark and Henneberg 2015, 2017, 2021a, 2021b). One of our papers was on the evolution of music and language. This study in the anatomy of the vocal tract was motivated by my love of music and my desire to see music become a more central component of our models of human evolution. That love, and the central role I attribute to music, ritual and dance in my understanding of human evolution, will become evident throughout this book.

An important note on terminology. I use the term hominin to refer to all of the species related to us that evolved over the last six to seven million years. Many of these species seem to have gone extinct, while others most likely contributed genetic material to modern human populations through interbreeding and gene flow. Sometimes, the term hominid is used to describe our lineage. I will not be using that term in my analysis. *Ardipithecus ramidus* is one of the earliest known fossils to possess uniquely hominin traits that distinguish our lineage from the two living species of chimpanzee that are our closest living genetic relatives – the common chimpanzee and the bonobo.

Current genetic evidence suggests that hominins shared a common ancestor with chimpanzees and bonobos some six to seven million years ago. During Jung's life, the majority of fossils that had been discovered were of *Homo erectus* and Neanderthal. These populations are quite recent in evolutionary terms and are very similar to modern humans in many ways. I use the term populations as opposed to species as it is not even clear if Neanderthals are a separate species from us or merely a populational variant of our own species. The field of paleogenomics has shown that modern humans contain Neanderthal DNA which means our ancestors bred with Neanderthals and that consequently they are most likely not a separate species. Jung was fascinated by *Homo erectus* and Neanderthal fossils. However, at the time he was writing, they were believed to be an intermediary between ourselves and the great apes. Based on this limited understanding, Jung referred to these fossils as 'ape man.'

In Chapters 2 and 4, I discuss Jung's interest in these fossils and his knowledge of them which was quite limited. A contemporary rapprochement between palaeoanthropology and analytical psychology requires updating Jung's ideas on fossil science in light of advances in the field that have occurred since his passing. In Chapter 4, I discuss these issues as well as consider possible ways of reconstructing the brain ontogeny of the much earlier hominins such as *Ardipithecus ramidus*. These early hominins most likely had a much shorter period of brain development and socio-cognitive maturation than we do – and also much shorter than *Homo erectus* and Neanderthals. In my attempt to update Jung's thinking, I apply his theory of the ontogenetic and phylogenetic emergence of consciousness to the much richer fossil record we now possess. In this context, his ideas are incredibly fruitful and seem to be consilient with some of the most recent research in evolutionary neuroscience.

One of the reasons Jung's evolutionary thought retains importance for contemporary understanding of human psychology is that his ideas were based on the comparative anatomical and evolutionary embryological approach of the Jena school and the *Naturphilosophen* (Clark 2023). While this tradition was overlooked during most of the twentieth century in recent decades, it has been reassessed by researchers in the field of evolutionary developmental biology or what has become known as Evo-Devo.

Evo-Devo investigates homologous (or archetypal) structures shared by a vast range of distantly related species. What researchers in this field have found is that many of the differences between living species are not so much due to differences in coding DNA but differences in genes that regulate the expression of coding DNA. In other words, such genes can alter development. Evo-Devo is in essence a modern form of research based on the relationship between ontogeny and phylogeny, and how underlying changes in the regulation and expression of homologous structures can lead to the diversification of species. Although Goethe and the *Naturphilosophen* lacked an understanding of genes, their theories based on anatomical archetypes have stood the test of time and have been verified by modern evolutionary genetics. Given this reassessment of the tradition out of which Jung's evolutionary thinking developed, it seems appropriate to reconsider the evolutionary basis of Jung's thought (Clark 2023).

The model of analytical psychology outlined in this book is based on current research in palaeoanthropology and evolutionary neuroscience. While I have biases in my interpretation of the fossil record, I have endeavoured to point out those biases by highlighting where issues of controversy still remain and alerting the reader to alterative perspectives in the literature. As is often the case in science, much is unsettled, and different researchers have differing views of the same data.

This is particularly the case in palaeoanthropology where we attempt to reconstruct the social and sexual behaviour of hominins that lived millions of years ago based on very scant fossil remains that have often been damaged by the ravages of time. Such uncertainty leaves a great deal of room for researchers to interpret the data in different ways according to prior assumptions. The result is a field rife with heated disputes and scholarly disagreement. Consequently, the research used in this book may very well be superseded in the future. However, I suspect that the general thesis will stand the test of time. In its broad outlines, I believe it reflects an aspect of truth about our species and our evolutionary emergence.

References

Alcaro, A., S. Carta, and J. Panksepp 2017. 'The Affective Core of the Self: A Neuro-Archetypical Perspective on the Foundations of Human (and Animal) Subjectivity', *Frontiers in Psychology*, 8: 1–13.

Bodkin, M. 1958. *Archetypal Patterns in Poetry: Psychological Studies of Imagination* (Vintage Books).

Carhart-Harris, R.L., and K.J. Friston 2010. 'The Default-Mode, Ego-Functions and Free-Energy: A Neurobiological Account of Freudian Ideas', *Brain*, 133: 1265–83.

Carhart-Harris, R.L., R. Leech, P.J. Hellyer, M. Shanahan, A. Feilding, E. Tagliazucchi, et al. 2014. 'The Entropic Brain: A Theory of Conscious States Informed by Neuroimaging Research with Psychedelic Drugs', *Frontiers in Human Neuroscience*, 8: 1–22.

Carter, C. S. 2022. 'Oxytocin and Love: Myths, Metaphors and Mysteries', *Comprehensive Psychoneuroendocrinology*, 9: 100107.

Clark, G. 2020a. 'Carl Jung, John Layard and Jordan Peterson: Assessing Theories of Human Social Evolution and Their Implications for Analytical Psychology', *International Journal of Jungian Studies*, 12: 129–58.

Clark, G. 2020b. 'Integrating the Archaic and the Modern: The Red Book, Visual Cognitive Modalities and the Neuroscience of Altered States of Consciousness.' in Stein, M., and T. Arzt (eds.), *Jung's Red Book for Our Time: Searching for Soul under Postmodern Conditions* (Chiron Publications).

Clark, G. 2021. 'Carl Jung and the Psychedelic Brain: An Evolutionary Model of Analytical Psychology Informed by Psychedelic Neuroscience', *International Journal of Jungian Studies*, 14(2): 1–30.

Clark, G. 2022. 'The Dionysian Primate: Goethe, Nietzsche, Jung and Psychedelic Neuroscience.' in Miils, J., and D. Burston (eds.), *Psychoanalysis and the Mind-Body Problem* (Rouledge).

Clark, G. 2023. 'Rethinking Jung's Reception of Kant and the Naturphilosophen: Archetypes, Evolutionary Developmental Biology and the Future of Analytical Psychology', *International Journal of Jungian Studies*, 1: 1–31.

Clark, G., and M. Henneberg. 2015. 'The Life History of Ardipithecus ramidus: A Heterochronic Model of Sexual and Social Maturation', *Anthropological Review*, 78: 109–32.

Clark, G., and M. Henneberg. 2017. 'Ardipithecus ramidus and the Evolution of Language and Singing: An Early Origin for Hominin Vocal Capability', *HOMO – Journal of Comparative Human Biology*, 68: 101–21.

Clark, G., and M. Henneberg. 2021a. 'Cognitive and Behavioral Modernity in Homo erectus: Skull Globularity and Hominin Brain Evolution', *Anthropological Review*, 84: 467–85.

Clark, G., and M. Henneberg. 2021b. 'Interpopulational Variation in Human Brain Size: Implications for Hominin Cognitive Phylogeny', *Anthropological Review*, 84: 405–29.

Dissanayake, E. 2021. 'Ancestral Human Mother-Infant Interaction Was an Adaptation that Gave Rise to Music and Dance', *Behavioral and Brain Sciences*, 44: e68.

Edinger, E.F. 1986. *Encounter with the Self: A Jungian Commentary on William Blake's Illustrations of the Book of Job* (Inner City Books).

Edinger, E.F. 1990. *Goethe's Faust: Notes for a Jungian Commentary* (Inner City Books).

Finnegan, M. 2013. 'The Politics of Eros: Ritual Dialogue and Egalitarianism in Three Central African Hunter-Gatherer Societies', *Journal of the Royal Anthropological Institute*, 19: 697–715.

Goodwyn, E.D. 2014. 'Depth Psychology and Symbolic Anthropology: Toward a Depth Sociology of Psychocultural Interaction', *The International Journal for the Psychology of Religion*, 24: 169–84.

Greenwood, S. 2013. 'Emile Durkheim and C. G. Jung: Structuring a Transpersonal Sociology of Religion', *International Journal of Transpersonal Studies*, 32: 42–52.

Hall, B.K. 1993. *Evolutionary Developmental Biology* (Springer Netherlands).

Harding, M.E. 1936. *Woman's Mysteries: Ancient and Modern* (Longman).

Haule, J.R. 2011a. *Jung in the 21st Century: Evolution and Archetype* (Routledge).

Haule, J.R. 2011b. *Jung in the 21st Century: Synchronicity and Science* (Routledge).

Jung, C.G. 1991. *Psychological Types* (Routledge).

Jung, C.G. 1992. *Two Essays on Analytical Psychology* (Routledge).

Kenny, A. 2013. *The Aranda's Pepa: An Introduction to Carl Strehlow's Masterpiece Die Aranda- und Loritja-Stämme in Zentral-Australien (1907-1920)* (ANU E Press).

Kimball, J. 1997. *Odyssey of the Psyche: Jungian Patterns in Joyce's Ulysses* (Southern Illinois University Press).

Knight, C. 1988. 'Menstrual Synchrony and the Australian Rainbow Snake.' in Buckley, T., and A. Gottlieb (eds.), *Blood Magic: The Anthropology of Menstruation* (University of California Press).

Knight, C. 1995. *Blood Relations: Menstruation and the Origins of Culture* (Yale University Press).

Knight, C., and J. Lewis 2016. 'Towards a Theory of Everything.' in Power, C., M. Finnegan, and H. Calla (eds.), *Human Origins: Contributions from Social Anthropology* (Berghahn Books).

Lawson, T.T. 2008. *Carl Jung, Darwin of the Mind* (Karnac).

Lewis-Williams, D., and S. Challis 2011. *Deciphering Ancient Minds: The Mystery of San Bushman Rock Art* (Thames & Hudson).

Mauss, M. 1910. 'Les Aranda et Loritja d'Australie centrale. I.', *L'Année sociologique*, 11: 76–81.

Mauss, M. 1913. 'Les Aranda et Loritja d'Australie centrale. II.', *L'Année sociologique*, 12: 101–4.

Morphy, H. 1997. 'Gillen: Man of Science.' in Mulvaney J., H. Morphy, and A. Petch (eds.), *'My Dear Spencer': The Letters of F. J. Gillen to Baldwin Spencer* (Hyland House).

Morphy, H. 1988. 'Spencer and Gillen in Durkheim: The Theoretical Constructions of Ethnography.' in Allen, N.J., W.S.F. Pickering, and W.W Miller (eds.), *On Durkheim's Elementary Forms of Religious Life* (Routledge).

Neumann, E. 1994. *The Fear of the Feminine: And Other Essays on Feminine Psychology* (Princeton University Press).

Nietzsche, F. 2002. *Nietzsche: Beyond Good and Evil: Prelude to a Philosophy of the Future* (Cambridge University Press).

Perera, S.B. 1981. *Descent to the Goddess: A Way of Initiation for Women* (Inner City Books).

Power, C., M. Finnegan, and H. Callan 2017. *Human Origins: Contributions from Social Anthropology* (Berghahn Books).

Power, C., V. Sommer, and I. Watts. 2013. 'The Seasonality Thermostat: Female Reproductive Synchrony and Male Behavior in Monkeys, Neanderthals, and Modern Humans', *PaleoAnthropology*, 2013: 33–60.

Rowland, S. 1999. *C.G. Jung and Literary Theory: The Challenge from Fiction* (Palgrave Macmillan UK).

Singer, J. 1986. *The Unholy Bible: Blake, Jung, and the Collective Unconscious* (Sigo Press).

Staude, J. 1976. 'From Depth Psychology to Depth Sociology: Freud, Jung, and Lévi-Strauss', *Theory and Society*, 3: 303–38.

Stevens, A. 1990. *Archetype: A Natural History of the Self* (Routledge).

Stevens, A. 2002. *Archetype Revisited: An Updated Natural History of the Self* (Brunner-Routledge).

Wilson, E.O. 1999. *Consilience: The Unity of Knowledge* (Vintage Books).

Chapter 1

Jung and the Condition of Modernity

Evolution, the *Naturphilosophen* and Evo-Devo

Introduction

In this chapter, I discuss the historical background of Jung's evolutionary thought. Jung's approach to human psychology was influenced by the works of Charles Darwin, whose ideas profoundly revolutionised humanity's self-understanding in the second half of the nineteenth century. However, the conception of human evolution he was exposed to was in many senses one that developed out of German, as opposed to Anglo-American traditions in biology. This tradition, which focussed on comparative anatomy and developmental embryology, can be traced back to Kant, Goethe and the *Naturphilosophen*. It was continued by Ernst Haeckel and the evolutionary embryologists of the late nineteenth and early twentieth centuries.

This tradition focussed on the role of developmental processes as the source of species diversity and evolutionary innovation – a relationship that was most famously encapsulated in Haeckel's 'biogenetic law' and the putative relationship between ontogeny (development) and phylogeny (evolution of species). When Darwin's works were popularised in Germany – most notably by Haeckel himself (Haeckel 1887) – they were fused with pre-Darwinian German biology. While this tradition was neglected for most of the twentieth century, recent developments in experimental and theoretical biology have led to a reappraisal of the *Naturphilosophen* and their emphasis on development and anatomical archetypes shared by a diverse range of species. Given the reappraisal of this tradition, which was so important in the genesis of Jung's evolutionary thought, a reconsideration of analytical psychology in the context of contemporary evolutionary science seems warranted.

Significantly, among the *Naturphilosophen*, the peculiarly modern dichotomisation between the arts and sciences was much less pronounced than it is today, with many of the major figures formulating developmental and evolutionary conceptions of art and literature. These were premised on the assumption that the emergence of consciousness out of a prior unconscious state produced a state of dissociation or loss of wholeness, with art being the means by which humans remediate such dissociation. Jung extended this interdisciplinary approach to art and science in the context of early twentieth-century evolutionary theory and fossil science.

DOI: 10.4324/9781032624549-2

An Evolutionary Critique of Modernity

Of his early years, Jung wrote that 'mentally my greatest adventure had been the study of Kant and Schopenhauer. The great news of the day was the work of Charles Darwin' (Jung 2014b: 213). During the late nineteenth century, Darwin's theory of evolution revolutionised debates about human origins, not only connecting humans with the rest of the animal kingdom, but also highlighting the immense temporal depth of life on earth. Such depth was becoming increasingly apparent as palaeontologists (scientists who study the fossil record) revealed the extent and antiquity of past geological epochs. This conception of temporal depth, the evidence of past epochs in current geological formations and the slow process of change or evolution over vast periods of time was famously articulated in Charles Lyell's *Principles of Geology*, published in three volumes in the 1830s. This was one of the major influences on Darwin's theory as outlined in his 1859 *On the Origins of Species*. Lyell had suggested to Darwin a conception of life's emergence on earth in terms of slow evolutionary processes, traces of which have been left in fossil assemblages in ancient geological strata (Darwin 2008: 74).

As we will see, both fossil science and a geological conception of the earth's history were important influences on Jung's evolutionary thought. Additionally, not only did these sciences inform his conception of brain evolution; they also provided him with the basic metaphors in which he would articulate that conception. For example, Jung conceived of the psyche in terms of geological and archaeological strata, with the unconscious and our ancient hominin and primate ancestors representing more ancient layers of the brain than more recently evolved structures (Jung 1989: 161, 2020: 202). This issue will be explored in greater detail in Chapter 2 where I discuss Jung's writings on primatology and palaeoanthropology.

Combined with developments in astronomy, which extended humankind's conception of space, evolutionary theory extended our conception of time into the realm of geological or 'deep time' (Gould 1987: 2). Not only was humanity an apparently insignificant species in a vast and indifferent universe. It was also a very recent arrival on the scene preceded by millions of years of organic evolution. It became increasingly apparent that the evidence for such vast temporal expanses lay beneath our feet in the form of ancient rocks and fossils and the various geological strata to which they belonged.

The revelation of such vast spatial and temporal dimensions to the world we inhabited had a profoundly destabilising effect on religious and philosophical notions that saw humanity as the centre of a divinely ordained universe. This is the intellectual background of Jung's thought. These ideas underpin the unique intellectual horizons that were opened up due to the growth of scientific rationality and experimental empiricism during the Enlightenment and beyond to our own times. They are some of the implicit assumptions of modernity.

While Jung accepted the findings of geology, palaeontology and evolutionary theory, he did not, however, reject the religious nature of human experience. Jung had great respect for the *numinous* nature of religious experience as articulated by Rudolph Otto (Jung 2014c: 104). In *The Idea of the Holy*, Otto analysed the non-rational aspects of religious experience which Mircea Eliade in *The Sacred and Profane* would later develop in his conception of *homo religiosis* (Otto 1957: 1; Eliade 1959: 15). While the orthodox designation of our species is *Homo sapiens*, I have particular sympathy for the taxonomic nomenclature *Homo religiosis*. And this is just as much an empirical issue as anything else. For example, the neurobiology of our species seems primed to produce religious states of consciousness, which are reported cross culturally and seem to be an evolved component of our neural architecture that is evident in ritual life and various techniques for altering consciousness. While other animals do seek to alter consciousness through the ingestion of mind-altering plants (Samorini 2002), the complex cultural elaboration of means for doing so through ritual, song, dance and the ingestion of psychoactive compounds seems to be a unique characteristic of humanity that distinguishes us from all other extant primate species. In this sense, we are the Dionysian Primate (Clark 2022).

Jung approached religion, as an inherent characteristic of our species, from the perspective of the evolutionary empiricist. Given it is a species typical phenomenon, just as spinning webs is typical of spiders, it is one that requires an evolutionary explanation. Consequently, Jung responded to the disenchantment that Max Weber (1864–1920) argued was characteristic of modernity (Jenkins 2000) by analysing such disenchantment from a psychological perspective informed by evolutionary theory. This is the rich paradox at the heart of Jung's thought: his solution to the desacralisation and disenchantment resulting from the development of scientific rationalism was to apply the methods of that very same rationalist approach to the dissociation he felt characterised the cultural malaise of modernity. In this sense, the growth of scientific consciousness over the past 300–400 years, and the abrogation of other non-rational *numinous* modes of experience that accompanied that project, could itself be a phenomenon open to scientific investigation.

Consequently, far from Jung being an anti-Enlightenment thinker as Hauke has suggested (Hauke 2000), I will argue that Jung's approach represents the continuation and fulfilment of the promises of Enlightenment rationality and its focus on detached observation and empirical verification. This project is one of the most important achievements of humankind's efforts to understand our place in the universe, with profound and far-reaching implications. For example, it led to the crucial distinction between subjective representations of the world and how the world exists in and of itself, a distinction central to Kant's critique of epistemology in *Critique of Pure Reason*, first published in 1781. This distinction is fundamental to modern scientific, empirical investigation, and it is one that Jung, influenced by Kant, placed at the heart of his theory of the psyche.

According to Jung, earlier cultural periods had tended to confuse subjective states with objective reality, with unconscious content being projected onto the external world. For example, in the Platonic writings of Plotinus (204–270 CE), experiences of the *numinous* (what we would today refer to today as altered states of consciousness) are considered to be a feature of the external world. This system was elaborated in his *Enneads* which focusses on the relevance of these rare but profoundly significant mystical experiences for the understanding of the mind and the universe.

Plotinus is a key figure in late antiquity who had a far-reaching impact on the consequent history of philosophy. Jung took a deep interest in these ancient thought systems, and along with Gnosticism and alchemy, they informed his psychological approach to cultural and historical analysis (Jung 1953; Edinger 1999a, 1999b; Jung and Segal 2013). For Jung, these ancient traditions had cultivated a domain of experience that had become increasingly uncommon in the modern period as consciousness refined and developed an ethos of rational abstraction. In this sense, modern, rationalist humans had lost contact with the evolutionary foundations of consciousness. Furthermore, they had in Jung's view very little awareness that such a process had occurred, producing not only a cultural condition of dissociation, but also a lack of awareness that such dissociation existed. Such a cultural process of 'splitting off the unconscious' in Jung's view produces an 'unbearable alienation of instinct' that is 'the source of endless error and confusion' (Jung 2014b: 137). It was analysing, and at the same time seeking to heal such dissociation at both the individual and cultural levels, that was the prime objective of analytical psychology.

In approaching the human mind from the point of view of modern empiricism and evolutionary science, far from rejecting the human relevance of the *numinous* and sacred dimensions of life, Jung saw them as core components of the phenomenology of the human mind. In this sense, they need to be part of any adequate and comprehensive account of human history and culture. Jung believed that such experiences most likely emanate from ancient evolutionary subcortical layers of the brain (Jung 1960: 270). And it is here where Jung's modern empirical and epistemological stance becomes apparent. The error of past epochs was to confuse such archaic psychic content with features of the external world. As Edinger writes:

> Plotinus' basic system is a magnificent philosophical fantasy of the structure of the universe. He was clearly an individual of extraordinary imagination and intuition. It is as though his intuitive gifts perceived the basic structure of the psyche, which he then read into the universe. Since, as Jung puts it, there was no epistemological criticism in those days, this unfolding fantasy can provide us with basic data in which the psyche is describing its own structure and nature, thus making the material relevant today.
>
> (Edinger 1999a: 99)

Jung argued that the lack of epistemological critique and the primacy of subjective fantasy was a crucial factor in ancient Greek mythological thought. As he writes, the 'activity of the early classical mind was in the highest degree artistic: the goal of its interest does not seem to have been how to understand the real world as objectively and accurately as possible, but how to adapt it aesthetically to subjective fantasies and expectations.' Commenting on the ancient Greek belief that the sun was thought of as the father of heaven and earth and the moon as a fruitful mother, he avers that there 'arose a picture of the universe which was completely removed from reality, but which corresponded exactly to man's subjective fantasies' (Jung 2014d: 21).

Jung adopted a similar approach in his analysis of alchemy, Gnosticism and hermetic traditions which he argued failed to adequately distinguish between subjective fantasies and the world of external objects, with objects becoming imbued with the content of such fantasies. Additionally, he juxtaposed such 'heretical' traditions like Gnosticism with orthodox Christianity and argued that such traditions were to culture as the dream is to the individual – that is unconscious counterparts of waking rational consciousness. Further, he argued that official suppression of such traditions amounted to a repression of the deeper aspects of the psyche from which religious experience emanates.

This analysis was to inform his conception of 'deep time' and ancient evolutionary layers in the psyche, which he argued were superseded by more recent layers associated with the emergence of the conscious ego or sense of self. Jung traced this process from our pre-human primate ancestors, through prehistory and antiquity, to the Enlightenment and the twentieth century. Jung's basic assertion was that human populations and entire cultural aggregations could become inordinately dissociated from a very important domain of experience. Such dissociation arose particularly in the modern period, according to Jung, along with the growth of science and the abstracted and detached manner in which rational consciousness interrogated the objective world.

Despite his respect for the religious domain of life, it is clear throughout his oeuvre that Jung is not interested in abandoning the scientific project of Enlightenment rationalism and the empirical investigation of human evolutionary origins. He wanted to understand the limitations of Enlightenment rationalism as a cultural and historical phenomenon, while also deepening and refining its empiricist approach to understanding the evolution of the human body, brain and social life. This would enable human culture, and its associated modes of conscious awareness, to move beyond the Enlightenment's limited rationalistic conception of mind, while also extending the range of the phenomena it investigated.

This extension of rationalist empiricism meant an expanded conception of the human mind that encompassed cultural practices such as yoga, Eastern contemplative traditions, Indigenous ritual and shamanism (Jung 1953: 101, 1970, 2012). Consequently, such non-Western modes of consciousness, when considered as objects of scientific study, help us develop conceptions of the human psyche that are not historically or culturally contingent but universal aspects of our evolved neurobiology. Jung had no intention of replacing scientific empiricism with prescientific or non-Western practices – his intention was to broaden the phenomena science seeks to explicate. As he writes, when commenting on Asian mediation practices, such as those contained in *The Secret of the Golden Flower*:

Western consciousness is by no means the only kind of consciousness there is; it is historically conditioned and geographically limited, and representative of only one part of mankind. The widening of consciousness ought not to proceed at the expense of the other kinds of consciousness.

(Jung 1953: 55)

It is clear from this comment that Jung was interested in a widening of con-sciousness – that is an expansion and deepening of human knowledge. But that expansion means going beyond the limited cultural horizons of the West and its rationalist empiricist ethos, while also extending that ethos to include other modes of consciousness. The implication here is not an abandonment of the scientific pro-ject, but a widening and deepening of its scope and subject matter.

The scientific paradigms that Jung utilised for such a project were evolutionary theory, developmental embryology and brain science – or what today we would call neuroscience. This enabled him to develop a scientifically grounded theory of human cultural development which focussed on the changing nature of rationalistic ego consciousness, its various historical transformations and how this uniquely hu-man form of cognition was in a dialectical and often antagonistic relationship with more ancient brain systems.

Among the richest of Jung's contributions to human knowledge was not only his analysis of the refinement and differentiation of consciousness during the period of modernity, but his articulation of an emerging new stage in the evolution of con-sciousness. This new stage could be described as our emergence out of or beyond the period of modernity and Enlightenment rationalism, a process in which we integrate the major scientific advances of the past 300 years with the aspects of the mind that period had neglected and effectively repressed.

In this sense, the evolution of consciousness as we move beyond modernity does not entail a postmodern inspired rejection of science as just another form of nar-rative discourse equal in epistemic veracity to all others. Such a development of consciousness entails an evolutionary account, grounded in brain science, of cul-tural change and transformation. In this sense, it offers a meta-perspective on those changes, one that sits outside of them with culture becoming an object of critical scientific investigation. And it is that perspective, which Jung argued analytical psychology provides, that represents the frontier of human scientific knowledge as it pertains to cultural and historical analysis.

To put the issue another way, we could think of the framework provided by analytical psychology as representing a new stage in human consciousness where we are no longer *in* the culture of rationalist modernity but have adopted a critical perspective outside or above it so to speak. It is the difference between being an unconscious and uncritical participant in a cultural milieu, and a self-conscious and detached critical observer of that milieu. In this sense, Jung's evolutionary concep-tion of the culture of modernity is an attempt to become liberated from its limiting conception of the human psyche.

This is a very different response to the Enlightenment and modernity than that developed by Jungian scholars inspired by poststructuralism and postmodern critiques of language and power (Hauke 2000; Rowland 2002; Rowland 2004; Gardner and Gray 2016). While such analyses concur with Jung in their critical appraisal of the limitations of Enlightenment rationalism, they depart dramatically from his approach in their wholesale rejection of the Enlightenment project and the virtues of objective scientific investigation – what Rowland has dismissively called Jung's 'drive to grand theory' and his imitation of 'Enlightenment grand narratives' (Rowland 2002: 139).

Such postmodern approaches represent a rejection of the major advances in knowledge over the past 300 years. They reduce the human drive for self-awareness, for knowledge of our origins, to an oppressive narrative structure that lacks any traction in regard to objective reality – a nihilistic framework that foregrounds critique of oppressive language structures while rejecting science and erasing ontology, essence and subjectivity (Mills 2017). Such an approach is one that is completely antithetical to Jung's intentions of developing an evolutionary conception of the psyche. Jung was a nuanced dialectical thinker who could simultaneously appreciate the virtues of cultural phenomena as well as their shortcomings. Unfortunately, the above authors seem to lack such dialectical nuance. While they have embraced Jung's critique of the Enlightenment and its rationalist excesses, they explicitly reject Jung's attempt to form a scientifically grounded biological conception of consciousness and its evolution.

Other Jungians however have sought to extend Jung's intention of developing an evolutionarily grounded conception of the psyche (Stevens 2002; Haule 2011a, 2011b; Goodwyn 2012; Clark 2020a, 2020b, 2021, 2022, 2023). The different conceptual orientations of Jungians who seek to develop the scientific basis of Jung's thinking, and those inspired by poststructuralism and postmodernism, are epitomised by contrasting Anthony Stevens' *Archetype Revisited: An Updated Natural History of the Self* (Stevens 2002) and Christopher Hauke's *Jung and the Postmodern: The Interpretation of Realities* (Hauke 2000).

Stevens adopts an evolutionary approach utilising data from infant development and ethology to argue against postmodern linguistic analysis and social science models based on the notion that the human mind is a *tabula rasa* or blank slate (Stevens 2002: 49–50). Such accounts deny the existence of an underlying universal or biologically based human nature that is characteristic of our species; consequently, such 'blank slate' perspectives assert that the mind is formed by external cultural factors (Barkow, Cosmides, and Tooby 1995: 24–33; Pinker 2003). Jung was explicitly opposed to this view; as he writes the 'psyche of the child in its preconscious state is anything but a *tabula rasa*; it is already preformed in a recognisably individual way, and is moreover equipped with all specifically human instincts, as well as with the a priori foundations of the higher functions' (Jung 2011: 348). Stevens follows Jung in rejecting a *tabula rasa* model of the mind. He also rejects the influence such thinking has had in recent Jungian scholarship, arguing for a rapprochement between analytical psychology and broader trends in the empirical sciences.

In contrast, Hauke rejects Enlightenment rationalism and the scientific approach of empirical measurement and experimental replication. While Hauke's analysis of Enlightenment rationalism is astute, it lacks a positive appraisal of the empirical scientific method and how it can be utilised to advance our understanding of the neuroevolutionary basis of consciousness. In contrast to Hauke, I suggest that the most sound and robust method for overcoming the epistemological and ontological shortcomings of Enlightenment rationality is to extend its methods into an analysis of the evolution of the brain and culture as Jung intended. If Enlightenment rationality did represent a negation and repression of other aspects of the psyche – and if this negation is a fact in the world – then one of the most fruitful methods of explicating and understanding it at our disposal is the scientific method.

Here, we need to distinguish between the scientific method as an epistemological stance that seeks to remove the attribution of subjective states of the mind or belief to external phenomena, and the use of such methods by culturally embedded human beings. Such human beings can be unconsciously biased by broader cultural influences and unpacked ideological assumptions – as Jungians inspired by postmodernism have amply demonstrated. But one of the most efficacious methods we have of overcoming such biases, paradoxically, is through further application of the scientific method. This approach also has the benefit of bringing analytical psychology into dialogue with broader trends in our contemporary scientifically oriented culture, in which neuroscience and human origins are issues of both academic and broader public interest.

In the neurosciences, for example, the error involved in the valorisation of reason characteristic of the Enlightenment has been shown to be based on an inaccurate account of the human mind. This approach has provided solid empirical evidence that reasoning requires the guidance of feeling and emotion conveyed by the body (Damasio 2008). Deep similarities or homologies between the brain systems and neurochemical pathways evident when comparing humans and other animals suggest a very ancient evolutionary basis for empathy, maternal care and morality, thereby undermining the illusion that we are disembodied rational creatures (Panksepp 2004, 2011; Preston 2013; de Waal 2016). These developments in evolutionary neuroscience have been referred to as the 'rise of affectivism' (Dukes et al. 2021). This research, in much the same way as Jung sought to, uses rational and empirical investigation to undermine the valorisation of rationality that characterises Enlightenment conceptions of human beings.

Hauke criticises what he calls the 'Enlightenment … tools of observation and measurement' which are, he writes 'designed to exclude or control external influences and to emphasise a few key variables, or conditions, which can then be studied in a repeatable fashion' (Hauke 2000: 241 and 47). This is a concise description of the scientific method, which Hauke sees as a vice not a virtue. His reason for doing so is that he conceives of the scientific method as being implicated in the values of Western culture more generally. In this sense, science, technology and economic activity 'abstracts and alienates human consciousness' (Hauke 2000: 241). While Hauke is analysing a real cultural phenomenon, he makes the mistake of conflating the scientific method itself with the ways in which it has been applied in certain cultural and historical contexts.

As intimated above, experimental neuroscience – which is predicated on detached observation, measurement and experimental replication – has undermined many of the cultural prejudices about the human mind that were part of the West's cultural inheritance. This indicates that the privileging of reason during the period of the Enlightenment is not inherently coupled to scientific empiricism. Even more compelling evidence that scientific empiricism is not inherently bound to a rationalist conception of mind, in which the perceiving subject is abstracted and alienated from objects, comes from neuroimaging of altered states of consciousness. This research includes investigation of the neurobiological substrates and alterations of neural architecture observed in, for example, Eastern mediation and contemplative practices as well as altered or enriched states of consciousness involving ego-dissolving mystical experiences (Griffiths et al. 2006; Carhart-Harris et al. 2014; Metzinger 2020). Significantly, such experiences have been found to undermine the representational fictions of an enduring Cartesian self characteristic of Enlightenment philosophy (Letheby and Gerrans 2017). Such approaches have also been able to elucidate the neural mechanisms underlying the transition from egoism to ecoism or nature connectedness, forms of non-dual awareness and various other states of mind in which the dualistic sense of distance between the mind and external reality is obviated (MacLean, Johnson, and Griffiths 2011; Josipovic 2013; Kettner et al. 2019).

Such research opens the possibility of integrating Eastern meditation and contemplative traditions, as well as cross-cultural ritualistic methods of altering consciousness, into a broader neurophenomenological conception of mind (Clark 2022). This unification of philosophy with such traditions is believed to offer 'considerable enrichment within analytical philosophy of mind itself, by elevating comparative and transcultural philosophy of mind to a new and more systematic level' (Metzinger 2020: 5). Jung, I suggest, was a pioneer of such a transcultural conception of mind.

This research provides empirically based methods of developing Jung's ideas in a manner that is consilient with major developments in contemporary science. And this is not based on an attempt to cleave Jung's ideas into paradigms where the fit is inappropriate or forced. What has happened is neuroscience has caught up with Jung, who, as an empirical phenomenologist of consciousness, was well aware of dimensions of human experience suppressed during the period of rationalist modernity. Now that experimental neuroscience is exploring those domains of experience that Jung spent his life researching, we can now appreciate that he was far ahead of his time and that science has a half a century after his passing begun to catch up with him.

Elsewhere, I have explored Jung's thoughts on the psychedelic research that was undertaken during 1950s and 1960s (Clark 2021). In that article, I sought to develop an approach to Jung grounded in psychedelic neuroscience. Significantly, while sceptical of their use – or misuse – Jung did seem to understand the nature of the psychedelic experience; as he writes: psychedelics 'lay bare a level of the unconscious that is otherwise accessible only under peculiar psychic conditions' giving rise to perceptions and experiences similar to those occurring 'either in mystical states or in the analysis of unconscious phenomena' (Jung, Adler, and Jaffé 1976: 382).

Modern research into the effects of these compounds shows that they do, as Jung suggested, produce mystical and numinous experiences – and quite reliably in laboratory settings (Griffiths et al. 2006). It has been argued that neurochemical modifications to the brain occasioned by ingestion of psychedelic compounds induce alterations in brain connectivity that correlate with archetypal religious experiences of 'ego dissolution' and 'oceanic boundlessness' (Kettner et al. 2019: 4; Carhart-Harris and Friston 2019: 317 and 336).

Given these findings, Jung's theories regarding the phenomenology of religious experience, and the emergence of unconscious material into consciousness awareness, seem to be consilient with findings in contemporary psychedelic neuroscience (Carhart-Harris et al. 2014; Clark 2021, 2022). Further, this research has produced evidence that such experiences have quite profound potential to heal mental suffering, effect dramatic positive changes in personality and significantly enrich and deepen personal meaning and well-being, particularly when used in the context of supportive psychotherapy (Griffiths et al. 2006, 2008; Carhart-Harris and Friston 2010; MacLean, Johnson, and Griffiths 2011; Clark 2021).

In Chapter 5, I will argue that such modes of consciousness, in the words of Benny Shanon, bring us to the 'boundaries not only of science but also of the entire Western world view and its philosophies' (Shanon 2002: 39). I would add the caveat that science has crossed those boundaries. We are now developing models of consciousness using empirically rigorous scientific methods that explore the deepest aspects of the psyche and the neurobiological font of archetypal religious experience.

When considering the debate between Stevens and Hauke noted above, I will argue that Stevens' position is more attractive as he defends the scientific method as opposed to rejecting it. There is also a lot to recommend his view that the rejection of evolutionary science by numerous Jungians is due to the fact that the 'biological roots of Jung's hypothesis' is seen 'as antipathetic to the liberal causes that neo-Jungians espouse—such as sexual and racial equality' (Stevens 2002: 69). I see no reason, however, why this should be so, given that numerous feminists accept biologically based differences between the sexes, and that evolutionary neurobiology can help illuminate the rich experiential nature of Indigenous ritual life and shamanic practices (Gowaty 1992, 2012; Winkelman 2010; Clark 2021, 2022; Stock 2023; Sullivan and Todd 2023). Nevertheless, Steven's diagnosis seems to be valid:

Instead of receiving a grounding in biology, most contemporary Jungians are products of university departments in which the standard social science [*tabula rasa*] model has continued to enjoy the status of holy writ. As a result, when they come to study Jungian theory, they are forced to reconcile what they have been taught to see as the extreme plasticity of human psychology with Jung's notion of an innately structured psyche. To resolve this paradox most feel a need to distance themselves from Jung's evolutionary perspective in order to redefine archetypal theory in a form compatible with the anti-biological consensus of the social sciences. The effect of this revisionist undertaking is to push analytical psychology back to the *tabula rasa* model which Jung so decisively rejected at the beginning of the twentieth century.

(Stevens 2002: 55)

Stevens avers that 'to persist in this misguided course is to sustain a self-inflicted wound of potentially fatal proportions. It could destroy the very foundations on which the entire Jungian edifice is built' (Stevens 2002: 55). In what follows, I explore these foundations – in terms of both their historical origin and areas of consilience between analytical psychology and major trends in contemporary scientific thought.

Jung, Evo-Devo and the *Naturphilosophen*

The version of evolutionary theory that Jung encountered would have been distinctively European or more specifically German. In the eighteenth and nineteenth centuries, a group of philosophers, scientists, artists and poets known as the *Naturphilosophen* formulated theories regarding anatomical archetypes that highlighted affinities between a diverse range of species. They also debated evidence for evolution prior to Darwin publishing his revolutionary *On the Origin of Species* in 1859. Noting the underlying anatomical affinities between a diverse array of species, combined with observation of changes in organic form throughout development, they speculated about similar transformations of organic form over geological time.

The *Naturphilosophen*, who included Johann Wolfgang von Goethe (1749–1832), Friedrich Schelling (1775–1884), Carl Gustav Carus (1789–1869) and Erst Haeckel (1834–1919), were a group of researchers and writers focussed around the University of Jena where a vibrant intellectual culture developed in which science, poetry and philosophy intermingled, with 'observation of nature' being 'cultivated both artistically and empirically' (Jahn 1994: 75). This group of thinkers provided many of the basic concepts that Jung adopted in his writings, from comparative anatomy and the relationship between ontogeny and phylogeny, to their conception of the unconscious as a creative and productive force that exists antecedent to consciousness (Clark 2023).

The notion of underlying osteological archetypes shared by a diverse array of species became a central premise of the comparative anatomical approach developed by members of the Jena school. It was this comparative anatomical approach that underpinned Jung's conception of deep archetypal affinities, in both the brain and body, that link humans to the vast array of other species we share the planet with (Clark 2023). Their theories of nature derived from observation of developmental processes in plants, animals and humans, noting how organismic change and transformation from the earliest stages of embryogenesis and throughout development result in the mature adult form. Such developmental conceptions derived from observation of nature were also applied to human psychology and theories of art. More specifically, this involved the notion that throughout human development, self-consciousness emerged out of a more primary state referred to as the unconscious. For the *Naturphilosophen*, art became a means of healing the division resulting from such developmental processes (Davis 2018). In this sense, studies of anatomy, developmental processes and art were integrated into a unified conception of nature and mind.

The role of the *Naturphilosophen* in the development of evolutionary theory is becoming increasingly recognised by historians of science. Most notably in his *The Romantic Conception of Life: Science and Philosophy in the Age of Goethe*, Robert Richards provides extensive evidence that German Romanticism and nineteenth-century German philosophy and biology had a significant impact on Darwin's thinking. As he writes, Darwin's nature, like that of the German Romantics, exemplified 'archetypal patterns beneath the wild frenzy of their variations' (Richards 2010: 52–54).

While Richards is not concerned with Jung, his book provides a rich account of the scientific and cultural background out of which Jung's ideas emerged. Scholars have explored in detail Jung's relationship to the Jena school and the *Naturphilosophen* in terms of literary and philosophical influence (Bishop 1996, 2000, 2007, 2008; Cambray 2013, 2017; Barentsen 2020), while less consideration has been given to the influence of the scientific theories of the *Naturphilosophen* on Jung's thought. Significantly, Cambray has suggested that developments in the biological sciences can inform the future of analytical psychology, noting that Jung's theories on the 'archaeological layering of the collective unconscious, with their Haeckelian overtones' could be explored in the context of contemporary evolutionary developmental biology and the recent reappraisal of the *Naturpohilosophen* (Cambray 2017: 43). Elsewhere, I have taken up Cambray's suggestion and explored in depth how the scientific theories of the *Naturphilosophen* informed Jung's evolutionary thought (Clark 2023).

As elaborated by Richards, Goethe was a major figure in this movement, and he wrote important studies on plant development as well as the anatomical affinities between humans and other animals (Goethe 1988; Goethe 2009). For example, in his essay *An Intermaxillary Bone is Present in the Upper Jaw of Man as Well as Animals* (1786), Goethe analysed the different degrees of differentiation of underlying osteological archetypes (Goethe 1988: 115 and 24). These affinities can be seen in Figure 1.1 where the existence of the premaxillary bone (that is the frontal portion of the upper jaw) is evident in both humans and horses. However, in humans, this bone and the associated structures of the face and jaw have been reduced dramatically relative to other animals – so much so that for centuries it had been assumed that humans lacked this distinctive feature of animal anatomy. It was the supposed absence of this bone that had underpinned the presumed separation

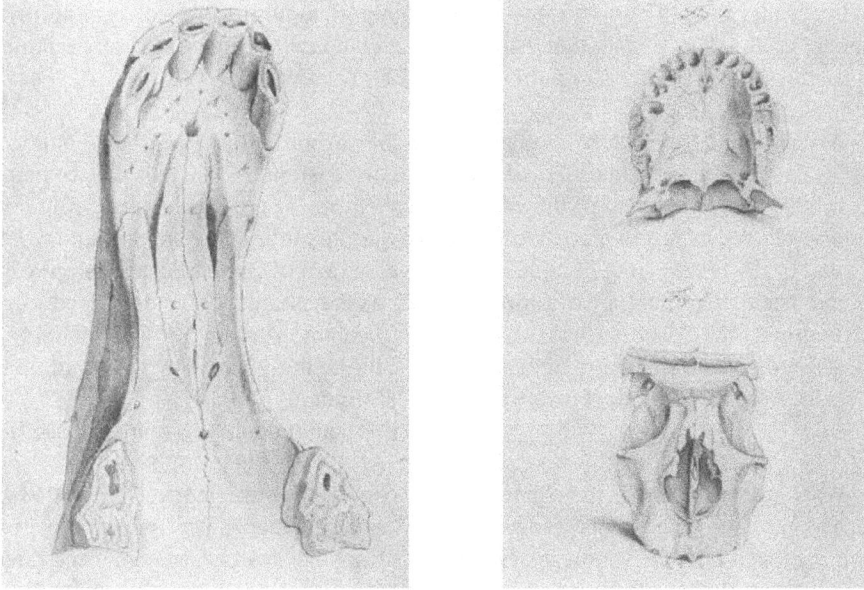

Figure 1.1 The upper jaw of a horse and human, from Goethe's *An Intermaxillary Bone is Present in the Upper Jaw of Man as Well as Animals* (1786). The intermaxillary bone is the long extended part of the jaw housing the front teeth in the horse (left). In the human jaw (right), it is greatly reduced but still evident. The suture or faint line across the top of the jaw is where the intermaxillary bone fuses with the rest of the jaw.

between humans and other animals – a separation which Goethe's studies undermined (Ashley-Montagu 1935).

What Goethe observed was that the premaxillary bone exists in human embryos and other animals – but that in humans as we mature, the premaxillary bone fuses with the rest of the jawbone (Goethe 1988: 111–6). It was the fusing of the premaxillary bone with the rest of the jaw that made it appear as if it did not exist in humans. Goethe's focus on embryology and development enabled him to perceive anatomical affinities between humans and other animals that had been previously overlooked. More specifically, it resulted in Goethe advancing the position that humans and other animals, and particularly the apes, were related due to possessing shared underlying anatomy (Richards 2010: 375). Importantly, during the nineteenth century, Goethe's theory of anatomical archetypes presented the most 'famous proposal among a set of archetypal theories that would soon sweep the world of animal morphology' (Gould 2002: 1092). Additionally, Goethe's theory of an underlying anatomical archetype or blueprint shared by a diverse range of species would be one of the major ideas of the period that paved the way for Darwin's theory of evolution (Gould 2002: 11; Richards 2010, 2013, 2017).

Immanuel Kant (1724–1804) was also an important figure who had a significant impact on the *Naturphilosophen* and German comparative anatomy. For example, in his *Critique of Judgement* published in 1790, Kant wrote:

> Many animal species resemble one another according to a certain common scheme, which scheme seems to lie at the foundation not only of the structure of their bones but also of the ordering of their other parts, so that the proliferation of species might arise according to a simple outline: the shortening of one part or the lengthening of another, the development of one part or the atrophy of another ... This analogy of forms—insofar as they seem to have been produced, despite their differences, according to common archetypes [*Urbilde*]—strengthens the suspicion of a real relationship of these forms by reason of their birth from a common, aboriginal mother [*Urmutter*].
>
> (Kant quoted in Richards 2000: 28)

What is at issue here is the connection between what Ernst Haeckel (1834–1919) was to later designate in his 'biogenetic law' as the relationship between ontogeny and phylogeny. In the simplest of terms, this theory states that changing the rates of growth during ontogeny can account for the different anatomical structures in a wide range of species. For example, the fins of fish, the limbs of lizards, the wings of birds and the hands of humans are similar in their anatomical structure and the composition of bones (Hall 2008). However, each represents a modification of this underlying shared archetypal structure with some bones growing more and some less. Consequently, phylogeny or speciation results from the alteration of ontogenetic growth trajectories. This variation on an underlying archetypal theme is what seems to account for species diversity.

While Haeckel's formulation of these concepts in his 'biogenetic law' is the most known today, he was merely giving expression to a widely held view on organic form. That view is evident in Kant's formulation above where altered rates of growth in the skeleton can produce different anatomical forms; as he stated 'the shortening of one part or the lengthening of another, the development of one part or the atrophy of another.'

A similar conception was proposed by the German biologist Carl Friedrich Kielmeyer (1765–1844) as early as 1793 in which he postulated a 'parallelism between stages of development and the series of living organisms' (Appel 1987: 107). Carus, an accomplished comparative anatomist, also developed an early formulation of the notion that ontogeny recapitulates phylogeny, as well as an embryological and development conception of psychology (Carus 1827; Ellenberger 1970; Bell 2010: 207; Carus 2017: 73–74). His comparison of the anatomical structures shared by a diverse range of species can be seen in Figure 1.2. While Jung's interest in the relationship between development and evolution has been attributed to the influence of Haeckel's 'biogenetic law' (Bair 2003: 215, 718 and 720), it is important to remember that Haeckel's conception was the formulation of an idea that had been developed by earlier thinkers.

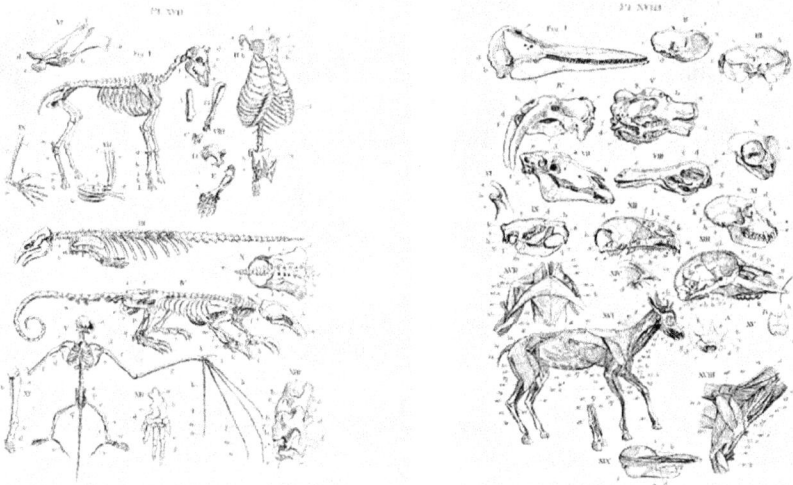

Figure 1.2 Shared anatomical structures from Carus' *Introduction to Comparative Anatomy: Twenty Plates* (1827), Plates XVII and XVIII.

While the *Naturphilosophen* speculated about alterations of development giving rise to new species, they also applied developmental perspectives to human psychology. This developmental approach, particularly in the work of Schelling and Carus, focussed on the psychological trajectory of consciousness emerging out of prior unconscious states – what Carus referred to as the *'primordial source of life'* (McGrath 2012: 1–7; Carus 2017: 83). Significantly, Jung acknowledged the parallels between his own ideas and those of Schelling and Carus. For example, he stated that Schelling's notion of the 'eternally unconscious' as the absolute ground of consciousness represents a precursor to the concept of the collective psyche (Jung 2014b: 515). He also suggested that Carus prefigured the concept of the unconscious that was to be later developed in modern scientific and medical psychology (Jung 2014a: 3). Importantly, the work of Carus is believed to provide the background for understanding the *Weltanschauung* that informed Jung's thinking, enabling us to see the historical roots of many of his ideas (Hillman 2017: 10).

Noting these affinities, it has been suggested that the Jungian conception of the unconscious has more affinity with pre-Freudian thinkers such as Schelling, Novalis and the German Romantics than it does with Freud's conception (Barentsen 2020; Clark 2023). Significantly, it has been argued that the Jungian notion of a collective, productive and creative unconscious that is oriented towards the future and which contains potentialities unrecognised by the ego can be traced back to Schelling (Rogers 2020: 6). It is worth noting that this developmental conception of the emergence of consciousness also informed the *Naturphilosophen's* theories of art in which the developmental process of consciousness emerging out of a prior unconscious state was believed to give rise to a dissociated condition which art remediates (Davis 2018: 92 and 95).

As already noted, the concept of anatomical archetypes, developed by Kant and the *Naturphilosophen*, provided crucial pieces of evidence for Darwin when he was formulating his theory. Darwin's understanding of archetypes came mostly from his reading of Richard Owen (1804–1892), a palaeontologist who developed his own concept of anatomical archetypes from his study of Carus, who, in turn, built upon the earlier work of Goethe and Kant (Richards 2018).

Owen wrote numerous works on cross-species archetypes or what he referred to as homologies most notably in his *On the Archetype and Homologies of the Vertebrate Skeleton* (1848) and *On the Nature of Limbs* (1849). Owen's ideas were central to Darwin's theory of natural selection. Darwin's innovation was to interpret the archetypal forms studied by the *Naturphilosophen* as the ancestral form from which a diverse range of species evolved – what is today referred to as the last common ancestor of a specific taxonomic group. Darwin also developed the embryological and developmental approach of the *Naturphilosophen*, suggesting that evolutionary innovations could potentially derive from alteration of shared embryonic form. As he writes when commenting on Owen's *On the Nature of Limbs*: 'I look at Owen's "Archetypes" as more than ideal, as a real representation as far as the most consummate skill & loftiest generalization can represent the parent form of the Vertebrate' (Ospovat 1995: 146). Connecting the concept of archetypes to embryology and development, Darwin wrote in a letter to T.H. Huxley in 1854: 'I should have thought that the archetype in imagination was always in some degree embryonic, and therefore capable [of] generally undergoing further development' (Darwin 1903: 73–74). Commenting on this aspect of Darwin's theory, Brian Hall writes:

> It was of course Charles Darwin, with his theory of descent from common ancestors, who provided the evolutionary insight into why groups of organisms share a common plan or morphological type: common ancestors not common archetypes 'explain' common ground plans. Descent from a common ancestor provides the explanation for unity of type and for homologous structures.
>
> (Hall 1993: 58)

Ernst Haeckel (1834–1919) was another important figure associated with the Jena school (Richards 2008: 30 and 34). Haeckel published many specialised scientific as well as popular works on evolution that combined the theories of Goethe, Lamarck and Darwin (Haeckel 1887). The development of evolutionary morphology in Jena, and specifically by Haeckel, acted as an important stimulus to the growth of embryological and evolutionary thinking in Germany and throughout the broader European culture during the latter half of the nineteenth and into the twentieth centuries (Hoßfeld and Olsson 2003; Hall 2011: 402). In addition to developing the most influential conception of the relationship between ontogeny and phylogeny (Haeckel 1887; Gould 1977), Haeckel also had a significant impact on the developmental of evolutionary embryology, an impact which continues to this day (Hoßfeld and Olsson 2003).

Significantly, in his 1871 *Descent of Man*, Darwin acknowledges his debt to Haeckel's theories linking development and evolution as important influences on his own thinking (Darwin 2004: 19 and 26–27). Haeckel's ideas also had a profound influence on developmental psychology in the twentieth century from Freud and Jung to Piaget (Bair 2003: 215, 718 and 20; Cambray 2017; Koops 2012, 2015; Clark 2023).

The influence of the tradition of comparative anatomy and embryology – developed by Kant, Goethe and Schelling and further elaborated by Carus and Haeckel – can be clearly seen in Jung's writings. As he writes, 'comparative anatomy and … evolution … show that the structure and function of the human body are the result of a series of embryonic mutations' with Jung arguing that the 'correspondence between ontogenesis and phylogenesis' may also apply to 'psychology' (Jung 2014d: 24). Drawing out the implications of evolutionarily conserved embryological processes and brain development, Jung writes that the '… brain is produced in each embryo in all its differentiated perfection, and when it starts functioning it will unfailingly produce the same results that have been produced innumerable times before in the ancestral line' (Jung 2014c: 480).

For Jung, this 'ancestral line' extends not only into the early stages of hominin evolution, but into the deep past, linking humans with the earliest life forms; for example, when discussing the relationship between the 'psychic organism' and the 'body,' he states that in '… its development and structure, it still preserves elements that connect it with the invertebrates and ultimately with the protozoa' (Jung 2014c: 204). It was this approach that formed the basis of Jung's theory of shared or archetypal brain structures in all humans, structures that also connect us with other animals. As noted above, these shared structures are referred to as homologies by biologists. However, homologies and archetypes are essentially the same phenomenon – that is, biological structures shared by a diverse range of species as a result of inheritance from a common ancestor. In Chapter 4, I discuss this issue in greater detail, highlighting how neuroscientific research into homologous brain systems we share with other animals can illuminate Jung's concept of archetypes and an evolutionarily layered psyche.

Throughout most of the twentieth century, the developmental and embryological theories of the *Naturphilosophen* were neglected. This was primarily a result of the focus on population genetics and changes in gene frequencies that was part of the twentieth-century modern synthesis in theoretical biology (Huxley 2010; Pigliucci and Muller 2010). While the modern synthesis represented a major advance in evolutionary theory, it did not give sufficient attention to embryological and developmental processes and how such processes may be implicated in evolutionary changes and speciation events over geological time. This situation has changed in recent decades with the advent of evolutionary development biology or Evo-Devo, a discipline that studies the way that embryological and developmental processes are altered by regulatory genes (Carroll 2012). It is such regulation of development or ontogeny that is believed to be a central component in evolutionary change or phylogeny. This has led researchers to advance the notion that the modern synthesis needs to be revised in light of such research – what has been called the extended evolutionary synthesis (Pigliucci and Muller 2010).

Importantly, as a result of the Evo-Devo revolution in the biological sciences, there has been a reappraisal of the comparative anatomical approach and evolutionary embryology developed by the Jena school and the *Naturpohilosophen* (Coen 1999; Richardson and Keuck 2002; Gould 2002; Laubichler and Maienschein 2007: 55–61; Olsson, Levit, and Hoßfeld 2017; Niklas and Kutschera 2017: 281–312). Commenting on the developmental approaches of the *Naturpohilosophen* and their relevance to current research paradigms, Crespi and Leach have argued that Evo-Devo arose from the joining of two research traditions: the 'century-old conceptualizations of how embryonic development has evolved, and recent discoveries of how genes orchestrate changes and variation in development' (Crespi and Leach 2016: 205).

One of the main reasons Jungian scholars have rejected, and failed to adequately develop, Jung's evolutionary conception of the psyche is the assumption that the theories of Haeckel and the German embryological tradition have been discredited by modern biology (Fordham 1957: 20 and 30; Otis 1994: 5; Shamdasani 2003: 266–7). In Chapter 2, I analyse the problems with this critique, highlighting how scholars have misunderstood and misrepresented Hackel's ideas and consequently Jung's use of them.

The above discussion indicates that many of the central ideas of Jung's emerged out of the tradition of *Naturphilosophie* – from comparative anatomy and embryology to the emergence of consciousness out of prior unconscious processes. His conception of art also echoes the theory of aesthetics developed by Goethe, Kant, Schelling and Carus (Clark 2023). For example, Jung suggests that art and poetry frequently involve activation of the collective unconscious which has been 'inherited in the anatomical structure of the brain' (Jung 1966: 80–81). This is essentially the same as Carus' approach to art and the unconscious noted above which he conceived of as an expression of the *primordial source of life*.

Shamdasani has argued that the cultural environment in the first two decades of the twentieth century was one of both oppressive societal confinement accompanied by attempts to overcome the limitations of such confinement. The consequence was experimentation and cross-pollination between science, psychology and the arts. As he writes, clear 'demarcations among literature, art, and psychology had not yet been set; writers and artists borrowed from psychologists, and vice versa.' Commenting on the cultural context of Jung's composition of *The Red Book*, Shamdasani writes:

> Within this cultural crisis Jung conceived of undertaking an extended process of self-experimentation, which resulted in *Liber Novus*, a work of psychology in a literary form. We stand today on the other side of a divide between psychology and literature. To consider *Liber Novus* today is to take up a work that could have emerged only before these separations had been firmly established. Its study helps us understand how the divide occurred.
>
> (Jung and Shamdasani 2009: 194)

While Shamdasani's point that Jung's fusion of literary form and science was part of twentieth-century cultural developments is valid to a degree, Jung was merely extending an impulse that was part of the much earlier cultural background of nineteenth-century Germany (Clark 2023). This is where the real deep affinities begin to emerge between Jung's thought and the *Naturphilosophen*; as noted above among the Jena school, a vibrant intellectual culture developed in which science, poetry and philosophy intermingled (Jahn 1994: 75). Jung's work could quite legitimately be seen as the culmination of interdisciplinary traditions in German thought that can be traced back to Goethe and Kant and which became manifest in the works of the *Naturphilosophen* (Clark 2023).

Jung's response to the conditions Shamdasani noted was unique and idiosyncratic. During his confrontation with the unconscious that resulted in *Liber Novus*, he penetrated the depths of the unconscious psyche, depths which modern rational consciousness had become inordinately dissociated or 'split off' from (Jung 2014b: 253–64). This was a widespread cultural malaise that had its origins in many factors, notably among them the Enlightenment and the Scientific Revolution that gave rise to the disenchanted condition of modernity. Jung's response in *Liber Novus* was a highly symbolic combination of visual art and literary text imbued with deep religious sentiment.

However, Jung was still in many ways a man of the Enlightenment. His major concern was to make sense of his descent into the unconscious in terms congruent with his own culture. He rejected the temptation to turn away from his own rationalist and scientific cultural inheritance and sought to make sense of his experience in terms of that inheritance. This approach was driven by a desire to communicate his experiences in a manner that was comprehensible and acceptable to modern forms of scientific consciousness and norms of epistemology. This meant developing a theory of the psyche grounded in what was at the time the latest research in evolutionary theory, palaeoanthropology, brain science and anthropology. Consilience is the term E.O. Wilson has used for such multidisciplinary approaches that unify the humanities and the sciences. Importantly, Wilson, one of the most influential evolutionary biologists of the twentieth century, has argued that Jung's theory of archetypes should be integrated into modern scientific accounts of culture and human origins (Wilson 1999: 85 and 238). It is hoped that this study contributes further to that process of integration.

Jung's decision to remain faithful to Enlightenment rationalism and epistemology, and to understand his confrontation with the unconscious in terms of the evolutionary science of his day, was a wise one. It has resulted in his ideas gaining more, not less relevance, as science advances (Stevens 2002; Haule 2011a, 2011b; Carhart-Harris et al. 2014; Bulkeley 2016; Alcaro, Carta, and Panksepp 2017; Clark 2020b, 2023; Clark 2021, 2022). Jung's approach represented a broad interdisciplinary engagement with the major trends of scientific thought of his times. Unfortunately, it is a project many modern Jungians have for the most part abandoned. This does a disservice to not only Jung but to the intellectual culture of our own age. Jung would have rejected the retreat from science Jungians inspired by poststructuralism and postmodernism have advocated in recent decades. Such an approach goes against the grain of his entire oeuvre and his intention to bring the abrogated aspects of the psyche into dialogue with modernity and modern empirical science. It is a betrayal of his legacy. I hope this book goes some way to countering that betrayal.

References

Alcaro, A., S. Carta, and J. Panksepp. 2017. 'The Affective Core of the Self: A Neuro-Archetypical Perspective on the Foundations of Human (and Animal) Subjectivity', *Frontiers in Psychology*, 8: 1–13.

Appel, T.A. 1987. *The Cuvier-Geoffroy Debate: French Biology in the Decades before Darwin* (Oxford University Press).

Ashley-Montagu, M.F. 1935. 'The Premaxilla in the Primates', *The Quarterly Review of Biology*, 10: 32–59.

Bair, D. 2003. *Jung: A Biography* (Little Brown).

Barentsen, G. 2020. *Romantic Metasubjectivity through Schelling and Jung: Rethinking the Romantic Subject* (Taylor & Francis).

Barkow, J.H., L. Cosmides, and J. Tooby 1995. *The Adapted Mind: Evolutionary Psychology and the Generation of Culture* (Oxford University Press).

Bell, M. 2010. 'Carl Gustav Carus and the Science of the Unconscious.' in Nicholls, A., and M. Liebscher (eds.), *Thinking the Unconscious: Nineteenth-Century German Thought* (Cambridge University Press).

Bishop, P. 2007. *Analytical Psychology and German Classical Aesthetics: Goethe, Schiller, and Jung, Volume 1: The Development of the Personality* (Taylor & Francis).

Bishop, P. 2008. *Analytical Psychology and German Classical Aesthetics: Goethe, Schiller, and Jung Volume 2: The Constellation of the Self* (Taylor & Francis).

Bishop, P. 1996. 'The Use of Kant in Jung's Early Psychological Works', *Journal of European Studies*, 26: 107–40.

Bishop, P. 2000. *Synchronicity and intellectual intuition in Kant, Swedenborg, and Jung. Volume 46 of Problems in Contemporary Philosophy* (E. Mellen Press).

Bulkeley, K. 2016. *Big Dreams: The Science of Dreaming and the Origins of Religion* (Oxford University Press).

Cambray, J. 2013. 'Romanticism and Revolution in Jung's Science.' in Jones, R.A. (ed.), *Jung and the Question of Science* (Routledge).

Cambray, J. 2017. 'The Red Book: Entrances and Exits.' in Kirsch, T., and G. Hogenson (eds.), *The Red Book: Reflections on CG Jung's Liber Novus* (Routledge).

Carhart-Harris, R.L., and K.J. Friston. 2010. 'The Default-Mode, Ego-Functions and Free-Energy: A Neurobiological Account of Freudian Ideas', *Brain*, 133: 1265–83.

Carhart-Harris, R.L., and K.J. Friston. 2019. 'REBUS and the Anarchic Brain: Toward a Unified Model of the Brain Action of Psychedelics', *Pharmacological Reviews*, 71: 316.

Carhart-Harris, R.L., R. Leech, P.J. Hellyer, M. Shanahan, A. Feilding, E. Tagliazucchi, et al. 2014. 'The Entropic Brain: A Theory of Conscious States Informed by Neuroimaging Research with Psychedelic Drugs', *Frontiers in Human Neuroscience*, 8: 1–22.

Carroll, S.B. 2012. *Endless Forms Most Beautiful: The New Science of Evo Devo and the Making of the Animal Kingdom* (Quercus).

Carus, C.G. 1827. *An Introduction to the Comparative Anatomy of Animals: Compiled with Constant Reference to Physiology, and Elucidated by Twenty Copper-Plates* (Longman, Rees, Orme, Brown, and Green).

Carus, C.G. 2017. *Psyche: On the Development of the Soul. The Unconscious* (Spring Publications).

Clark, G. 2020a. 'Carl Jung, John Layard and Jordan Peterson: Assessing Theories of Human Social Evolution and Their Implications for Analytical Psychology', *International Journal of Jungian Studies*, 12: 129–58.

Clark, G. 2020b. 'Integrating the Archaic and the Modern: The Red Book, Visual Cognitive Modalities and the Neuroscience of Altered States of Consciousness.' in Stein, M., and T. Arzt (eds.), *Jung's Red Book for Our Time: Searching for Soul under Postmodern Conditions* (Chiron Publications).

Clark, G. 2021. 'Carl Jung and the Psychedelic Brain: An Evolutionary Model of Analytical Psychology Informed by Psychedelic Neuroscience', *International Journal of Jungian Studies*, 14(2): 1–30.

Clark, G. 2022. 'The Dionysian Primate: Goethe, Nietzsche, Jung and Psychedelic Neuroscience.' in Miils, J., and D. Burston (eds.), *Psychoanalysis and the Mind-Body Problem* (Rouledge).

Clark, G. 2023. 'Rethinking Jung's Reception of Kant and the Naturphilosophen: Archetypes, Evolutionary Developmental Biology and the Future of Analytical Psychology', *International Journal of Jungian Studies*, 1: 1–31.

Coen, E. 1999. *The Art of Genes: How Organisms Make Themselves* (OUP).

Crespi, B., and E. Leach. 2016. 'The Evolutionary Biology of Human Neurodevelopment.' in Boughner, J.C., and C. Rolian (eds.), Developmental Approaches to Human Evolution (John Wiley & Sons).

Damasio, A. 2008. *Descartes' Error: Emotion, Reason and the Human Brain* (Random House).

Darwin, C. 1903. *More Letters of Charles Darwin: A Record of His Work in a Series of Hitherto Unpublished Letters* (D. Appleton).

Darwin, C. 2004. *The Descent of Man, and Selection in Relation to Sex* (Penguin).

Darwin, C. 2008. *On the Origin of Species* (OUP).

Davis, W.S. 2018. *Romanticism, Hellenism, and the Philosophy of Nature* (Springer International Publishing).

de Waal, F. 2016. *Primates and Philosophers: How Morality Evolved* (Princeton University Press).

Dukes, D., K. Abrams, R. Adolphs, M. Ahmed, A. Beatty, and K. Berridge, et al. 2021. 'The Rise of Affectivism', *Nature Human Behaviour*, 5: 816–20.

Edinger, E.F. 1999a. *The Psyche in Antiquity: Early Greek Philosophy from Thales to Plotinus* (Inner City Books).

Edinger, E.F. 1999b. *The Psyche in Antiquity: Gnosticism and Early Christianity* (Inner City Books).

Eliade, M. 1959. *The Sacred and the Profane: The Nature of Religion* (Harcourt, Brace).

Ellenberger, H.F. 1970. *The Discovery of the Unconscious: The History and Evolution of Dynamic Psychiatry* (Basic Books).

Fordham, M. 1957. *New Developments in Analytical Psychology* (Routledge and K. Paul).

Gardner, L., and F. Gray. 2016. *Feminist Views from Somewhere: Post-Jungian Themes in Feminist Theory* (Taylor & Francis).

Goethe, J.W. 1988. *Scientific Studies* (Suhrkamp).

Goethe, J.W. 2009. *The Metamorphosis of Plants* (MIT Press).

Goodwyn, E.D. 2012. *The Neurobiology of the Gods: How Brain Physiology Shapes the Recurrent Imagery of Myth and Dreams* (Routledge).

Gould, S.J. 1977. *Ontogeny and Phylogeny* (Belknap Press of Harvard University Press).

Gould, S.J. 1987. *Time's Arrow, Time's Cycle* (Harvard University Press).

Gould, S.J. 2002. *The Structure of Evolutionary Theory* (Harvard University Press).

Gowaty, P.A. 1992. 'Evolutionary Biology and Feminism', *Human Nature*, 3: 217–49.

Gowaty, P.A. 2012. *Feminism and Evolutionary Biology: Boundaries, Intersections and Frontiers* (Springer Science & Business Media).

Griffiths, R.R., W.A. Richards, U. McCann, and R. Jesse. 2006. 'Psilocybin Can Occasion Mystical-Type Experiences Having Substantial and Sustained Personal Meaning and Spiritual Significance', *Psychopharmacology (Berl)*, 187: 268–83; discussion 84–92.

Griffiths, R.R., W.A. Richards, M.W. Johnson, U.D. McCann, and R. Jesse. 2008. 'Mystical-Type Experiences Occasioned by Psilocybin Mediate the Attribution of Personal Meaning and Spiritual Significance 14 Months Later', *Journal of Psychopharmacology*, 22: 621–32.

Haeckel, E. 1887. *The History of Creation, or, the Development of the Earth and Its Inhabitants by the Action of Natural Causes: A Popular Exposition of the Doctrine of Evolution in General, and of that of Darwin, Goethe, and Lamarck in Particular* (D. Appleton).

Hall, B.K. 1993. *Evolutionary Developmental Biology* (Springer Netherlands).

Hall, B.K. 2008. *Fins into Limbs: Evolution, Development, and Transformation* (University of Chicago Press).

Hall, B.K. 2011. *Ontogeny does not Recapitulate Phylogeny, It Creates Phylogeny: A Review of The Tragic Sense of Life: Ernst Haeckel and the Struggle over Evolutionary Thought, by Robert J. Richards* (Wiley Online Library).

Hauke, C. 2000. *Jung and the Postmodern: The Interpretation of Realities* (Routledge).

Haule, J.R. 2011a. *Jung in the 21st Century: Evolution and Archetype* (Routledge).

Haule, J.R. 2011b. *Jung in the 21st Century: Synchronicity and Science* (Routledge).

Hillman, J. 2017. 'Introduction.' in *Psyche: On the Development of the Soul. The Unconscious* (Spring Publications).

Hoßfeld, Uwe, and L. Olsson. 2003. 'The Road from Haeckel: The Jena Tradition in Evolutionary Morphology and the Origins of "Evo-Devo"', *Biology and Philosophy*, 18: 285–307.

Huxley, J.S. 2010. *Evolution, The Definitive Edition: The Modern Synthesis* (MIT Press).

Jahn, I. 1994. 'On the Origin of Romantic Biology and Its Further Development at the University of Jena between 1790 and 1850.' in Stefano, P., and M. Bossi (eds.), *Romanticism in Science: Science in Europe, 1790–1840* (Springer Netherlands).

Jenkins, R. 2000. 'Disenchantment, Enchantment and Re-Enchantment: Max Weber at the Millennium', *Max Weber Studies*, 1: 11–32.

Josipovic, Z. 2013. 'Neural Correlates of Nondual Awareness in Meditation', *Annals of the New York Academy of Sciences*, 1307: 9–18.

Jung, C.G. 1953. *Collected Works of C. G. Jung, Volume 13: Alchemical Studies* (Princeton University Press).

Jung, C.G. 1960. *The Collected Works of C.G. Jung: The Psychogenesis of Mental Disease* (Routledge & Kegan Paul).

Jung, C.G. 1966. *The Collected Works of C. G. Jung: The Spirit in Man, Art, and Literature* (Pantheon Books).

Jung, C.G. 1970. *Psychology and Religion: West and East* (Routledge).

Jung, C.G. 1989. *Memories, Dreams, Reflections* (Knopf Doubleday Publishing Group).

Jung, C.G. 2011. *Memories, Dreams, Reflections* (Knopf Doubleday Publishing Group).

Jung, C.G. 2012. *The Psychology of Kundalini Yoga: Notes of the Seminar Given in 1932* (Princeton University Press).

Jung, C.G. 2014a. *Collected Works of C.G. Jung, Volume 9 (Part 1): Archetypes and the Collective Unconscious* (Princeton University Press).

Jung, C.G. 2014b. *Collected Works of C.G. Jung, Volume 18: The Symbolic Life: Miscellaneous Writings* (Princeton University Press).

Jung, C.G. 2014c. *The Structure and Dynamics of the Psyche* (Taylor & Francis).

Jung, C.G. 2014d. *Symbols of Transformation* (Taylor & Francis).

Jung, C.G. 2020. *C.G. Jung Speaking: Interviews and Encounters* (Princeton University Press).

Jung, C.G., G. Adler, and A. Jaffé. 1976. *Letters* (Routledge).

Jung, C.G., and R. Segal. 2013. *The Gnostic Jung: Including Seven Sermons to the Dead* (Taylor & Francis).

Jung, C.G., and S. Shamdasani. 2009. *Liber Novus* (W.W. Norton & Company).

Kettner, H., S. Gandy, E.C.H.M. Haijen, and R.L. Carhart-Harris. 2019. 'From Egoism to Ecoism: Psychedelics Increase Nature Relatedness in a State-Mediated and Context-Dependent Manner', *International Journal of Environmental Research and Public Health*, 16: 5147.

Koops, W. 2012. 'Jean Jacques Rousseau, Modern Developmental Psychology, and Education', *European Journal of Developmental Psychology*, 9: 46–56.

Koops, W. 2015. 'No Developmental Psychology without Recapitulation Theory', *European Journal of Developmental Psychology*, 12: 630–9.

Laubichler, M.D., and J. Maienschein. 2007. *From Embryology to Evo-Devo: A History of Developmental Evolution* (MIT Press).

Letheby, Chris, and Philip Gerrans. 2017. 'Self Unbound: Ego Dissolution in Psychedelic Experience', *Neuroscience of Consciousness*, 1: 1–11.

MacLean, K.A., M.W. Johnson, and R.R. Griffiths. 2011. 'Mystical Experiences Occasioned by the Hallucinogen Psilocybin Lead to Increases in the Personality Domain of Openness', *Journal of Psychopharmacology*, 25: 1453–61.

McGrath, S. 2012. *The Dark Ground of Spirit: Schelling and the Unconscious* (Routledge).

Metzinger, T. 2020. 'Minimal Phenomenal Experience: Meditation, Tonic Alertness, and the Phenomenology of "Pure" Consciousness', *Philosophy and the Mind Sciences*, 1: 1–44.

Mills, J. 2017. 'Challenging Relational Psychoanalysis: A Critique of Postmodernism and Analyst Self-Disclosure', *Psychoanalytic Perspectives*, 14: 313–35.

Niklas, K.J., and U. Kutschera. 2017. 'From Goethe's Plant Archetype via Haeckel's Biogenetic Law to Plant Evo-Devo 2016', *Theory in Biosciences*, 136: 49–57.

Olsson, L., G.S. Levit, and U. Hoßfeld. 2017. 'The "Biogenetic Law" in Zoology: From Ernst Haeckel's Formulation to Current Approaches', *Theory in Biosciences*, 136: 19–29.

Ospovat, D. 1995. *The Development of Darwin's Theory: Natural History, Natural Theology, and Natural Selection, 1838-1859* (Cambridge University Press).

Otis, L. 1994. *Organic Memory: History and the Body in the Late Nineteenth & Early Twentieth Centuries* (University of Nebraska Press).

Otto, R. 1957. *The Idea of the Holy: an Inquiry into the Non-Rational Factor in the Idea of the Divine and Its Relation to the Rational* (Oxford University Press).

Panksepp, J. 2004. *Affective Neuroscience: The Foundations of Human and Animal Emotions* (Oxford University Press).

Panksepp, J. 2011. 'Cross-Species Affective Neuroscience Decoding of the Primal Affective Experiences of Humans and Related Animals', *PLOS ONE*, 6: e21236–e36.

Pigliucci, M., and G.B. Muller. 2010. *Evolution, the Extended Synthesis* (MIT Press).

Pinker, S. 2003. *The Blank Slate: The Modern Denial of Human Nature* (Penguin Books Limited).

Preston, S.D. 2013. 'The Origins of Altruism in Offspring Care', *Psychological Bulletin*, 139: 1305.

Richards, R.J. 2018. 'The Foundations of Archetype Theory in Evolutionary Biology: Kant, Goethe, and Carus', *Republic of Letters*, 6(1): 1–12.

Richards, R.J. 2000. 'Kant and Blumenbach on the Bildungstrieb: A Historical Misunderstanding', *Studies in History and Philosophy of Science Part C: Studies in History and Philosophy of Biological and Biomedical Sciences*, 31: 11–32.

Richards, R.J. 2008. *The Tragic Sense of Life: Ernst Haeckel and the Struggle over Evolutionary Thought* (University of Chicago Press).

Richards, R.J. 2010. *The Romantic Conception of Life: Science and Philosophy in the Age of Goethe* (University of Chicago Press).

Richards, R.J. 2013. 'The Impact of German Idealism and Romanticism on Biology in the Nineteenth Century.' in Ameriks, K. (ed.), *The Impact of Idealism: The Legacy of Post-Kantian German Thought: Volume 1: Philosophy and Natural Sciences* (Cambridge University Press).

Richards, R.J. 2017. 'Did Goethe and Schelling Endorse Species Evolution?' Chapter 9 in Faflak, J (ed.), *Marking Time: Romanticism and Evolution* (University of Toronto Press): 219–38.

Richardson, M.K., and G. Keuck. 2002. 'Haeckel's ABC of Evolution and Development', *Biological Reviews of the Cambridge Philosophical Society*, 77: 495–528.

Rogers, C.D. 2020. 'Psychoanalyzing Nature, Dark Ground of Spirit', *Journal of the Pacific Association for the Continental Tradition*, 3: 1–19.

Rowland, S. 2004. 'Jung's Ghost Stories: Jung for Literary Theory in Feminism, Poststructuralism, and Postmodernism.' in Baumlin, J., T., Baumlin, and G. Jensen (eds.), *Post-Jungian Criticism: Theory and Practice* (State University of New York Press).

Rowland, S. 2002. *Jung: A Feminist Revision* (Wiley).

Samorini, G. 2002. *Animals and Psychedelics: The Natural World and the Instinct to Alter Consciousness* (Inner Traditions/Bear).

Shamdasani, S. 2003. *Jung and the Making of Modern Psychology: The Dream of a Science* (Cambridge University Press).

Shanon, B. 2002. *The Antipodes of the Mind: Charting the Phenomenology of the Ayahuasca Experience* (Oxford University Press).

Stevens, A. 2002. *Archetype Revisited: An Updated Natural History of the Self* (Brunner-Routledge).

Stock, K. 2023. 'Is Womanhood a Social Fact?' in Todd, S., and A. Sullivan (eds.), *Sex and Gender: A Contemporary Reader* (Routledge).

Sullivan, A., and S. Todd. (eds.). 2023. 'Introduction.' *Sex and Gender: A Contemporary Reader* (Routledge).

Wilson, E.O. 1999. *Consilience: The Unity of Knowledge* (Vintage Books).

Winkelman, M. 2010. *Shamanism: A Biopsychosocial Paradigm of Consciousness and Healing* (Praeger).

Chapter 2

Fossils, Anthropology and Hominin Brain Phylogeny

Introduction

In the previous chapter, I discussed the historical and cultural contexts out of which Jung's ideas developed. One of the main points of that chapter was to highlight how Jung's ideas on organismic development and comparative anatomy informed his theories on the emergence of consciousness out of a prior unconscious state. This conception of the human mind, I suggested, links Jung's ideas to the *Naturphilosophen* and the German biological traditions which he would have become familiar with in his youth and during his early education.

During his formative years, Jung also took an interest in the fossil discoveries of the time – for example, the skulls of *Homo erectus* and Neanderthals that had been recently excavated in Asia and Europe and which provided some of the first fossil evidence of archaic hominins. These were exciting and revolutionary discoveries that began to lift the veil from the past – a veil that had long occluded humanity's knowledge of its own origins. At last, science began to reconstruct our origins as a species and to address questions that had engaged thinkers for thousands of years: what is the nature of life, what exactly are human beings and what is the nature of our relationship to other animals and the rest of the natural world?

These discoveries enabled Jung to begin thinking about conceptions of the mind, which he encountered in the works of the *Naturphilosophen*, in light of the emerging science of palaeoanthropology. This gave his thinking a temporal dimension that was unavailable to earlier thinkers like Goethe, Schelling and Carus. However, Jung's ideas about fossil science were essentially the same as those of the *Naturphilosophen* – in fact, it could be argued that he applied the ideas of the *Naturphilosophen* to his interpretation of the fossil record. Essentially, this is what Jung did in his theory of the ontogeny and phylogeny of consciousness, giving the ideas of the Jena school a sense of temporal depth they tended to lack, particularly among the earlier figures like Goethe, Schelling and Carus.

The other important strand in Jung's thinking was his engagement with the emerging science of anthropology. During the nineteenth and early twentieth centuries, scientists sought to reconstruct our prehistoric hunter-gatherer past by

DOI: 10.4324/9781032624549-3

studying living hunter-gatherer peoples, who were presumed to resemble our Pleistocene ancestors more than modern Europeans did. While this project was at times misguided in some of its assumptions, it produced a vast body of literature that opened up the past to science in ways previously unimagined.

Crucial to this project were Australian works of ethnography by Baldwin Spencer (1860–1929) and Francis Gillen (1855–1912). These works revolutionised European thought at the turn of the twentieth century, laying the foundations for modern ethnographic field work, studies of kinship and of Indigenous religion (Morphy 1988, 1997). Their works became important source texts for the emerging discipline of sociology, forming the basis of Durkheim's theory of elementary religious forms (Durkheim 2008) as well as being important influences on Sir James Frazer and Freud (Morphy 1997: 25–8; Freud 2012: 132–6). They were also a key source text for Jung's writings on ritual, totemism, sacred stones and the Indigenous creative period or what has become known as the Dreaming.

Jung's reading in anthropology provided him with extensive data to further elaborate on his evolving conception of human psychology. And it is with this reading that the various threads of his thinking seem to have come together; his understanding of the unconscious and comparative anatomy derived from the *Naturphilosophen*, the putative parallels between ontogeny and phylogeny, and the use of ethnographic data to explore possible prehistoric forms of consciousness, social organisation, kinship systems and ritual life.

Comparative Anatomy and Palaeoanthropology: Jung, Hominin Fossils and Deep Time

Jung's dream recounted in *Memories, Dreams, Reflections* of descending the successive levels or stories of a house has become famous for illustrating how the intimate nature of a personal dream influenced the trajectory of Jung's consequent intellectual development. That dream, according to Jung, symbolised 'a history of successive layers of consciousness' (Jung 1989: 161). The dream seems to have reawakened Jung's 'old interest in archaeology,' while also motivating him to begin reading mythology in order to better understand 'primitive' cultures and 'mankind's collective inheritance' (Shamdasani 2003: 295).

While this aspect of the dream is well known, what is less frequently noted are the associations with palaeoanthropology and the fossil discoveries of the period Jung came across in the lowest level beneath the house. After descending through various historical layers of the building, Jung came upon the deepest and oldest layer:

My interest by now was intense. I looked more closely at the floor. It was of stone slabs, and in one of these I discovered a ring. When I pulled it, the stone slab lifted, and again I saw a stairway of narrow stone steps leading down into the depths. These, too, I descended, and entered a low cave cut into the rock.

Thick dust lay on the floor, and in the dust were scattered bones and broken pottery, like remains of a primitive culture. I discovered two human skulls, obviously very old and half disintegrated. Then I awoke.

(Jung 1989: 159)

When Jung was a student, he worked as an assistant in the Anatomical Institute at Basel University. Significantly, it was his familiarity with the fossils of early humans at this time that seems to have formed the associations with the skulls in the dream. And it is at this time that his interest in comparative anatomy and palaeoanthropology seems to have merged. As he was to later write:

My then historical interests had developed from my original preoccupation with comparative anatomy and paleontology when I worked as an assistant at the Anatomical Institute. I was fascinated by the bones of fossil man, particularly by the much discussed *Neanderthalensis* and the still more controversial skull of Dubois' *Pithecanthropus*. As a matter of fact, these were my real associations to the dream.

(Jung 2014b: 214)

Pithecanthropus erectus was the name given to a skull found in 1891 on the island of Java in Indonesia by the Dutch paleoanthropologist Eugene Dubois (1858–1940). During the period Jung was writing, it was considered closer to apes than humans – a kind of intermediate 'ape man.' Since then, more evidence has come forth and it has been reclassified as a member of our own genus and is now part of the group called *Homo erectus* (Mayr 1963: 341). The same is the case with Neanderthals with one of the most fascinating findings of modern times being evidence of Neanderthal DNA in modern humans (Pääbo 2014). This suggests that these early hominins were much closer to modern humans than previously thought. However, as was common at the time, Jung referred to *Pithecanthropus* and Neanderthals as examples of 'ape man' (Jung 1970: 212–13, 1998: 1194–5). In Chapter 4, I discuss these issues in more detail when I consider the relationship of Jung's thought to contemporary palaeoanthropology in more detail.

Jung also connected psychology with geology in his analysis of past epochs. For example, he linked *Pithecanthropus* (*Homo erectus*) to his conception of geological time – that is the temporal expanse of deep time. For example, when discussing 'writing' and 'civilization' – which he avers emerged only in the last 5,000 or 6,000 years – Jung states that such recent cultural achievements do not 'form a decent geological layer.' Prior to these recent historical periods are however 'long ages of primitiveness.' While admitting that the *Homo erectus* and Neanderthal fossils had not been securely dated at the time, he nevertheless writes that 'Sinanthropos man' (another *Homo erectus* fossil) and 'the Neanderthal race ... are immensely old, because the anatomical features have changed considerably since.' Jung goes on to contrast the psychology of these early varieties of hominin – what he designates the 'old man' or 'ape man' – with modern forms of consciousness (Jung 1998: 1194–5).

In the following quote, Jung elaborates on how he conceives of the relationship between ancestral conditions, such as those mentioned above in relation to fossil hominins, and modern consciousness. When considered in relation to his conception of an evolutionarily layered psyche, we can see how Jung linked his psychological theory to archaic hominins and the fossils he had encountered in his dream. These represent the ancestral preconditions of modern consciousness:

> In so far as no man is born totally new, but continually repeats the stage of development last reached by the species, he contains unconsciously, as an a priori datum, the entire psychic structure developed both upwards and downwards by his ancestors in the course of the ages ... The conscious mind thinks as a rule without regard to ancestral preconditions and without taking into account the influence this a priori factor has on the shaping of the individual's fate. Whereas we think in periods of years, the unconscious thinks and lives in terms of millennia. We are still living in a wonderful new world where man thinks himself astonishingly new and "modern." This is unmistakable proof of the youthfulness of human consciousness, which has not yet grown aware of its historical antecedents.
>
> (Jung 2014a: 279–80)

We can see here how the various strands of Jung's thought began to crystallise, and how the developmental and embryological traditions of the *Naturphilosophen* were synthesised with his interest in fossil science and anthropology. The result was an evolutionary conception of human cultural and historical processes based on a dialectic between two distinct brain systems: one of a collective nature with deep roots in our primate and mammalian past and which is universally present among all members of *Homo sapiens*, the other a more recent evolutionary innovation involving the emergence of individualised ego consciousness.

This more recent brain system could give rise to rapid changes in culture, thereby accounting for differences between, for example, modern industrial societies and those of hunter-gatherer societies; as Lawson avers within the last 6,000 years, the 'rapid, evolution of consciousness can be charted in developments in civilizations through history' (Lawson 2008: 4). That more recent system of self-reflective ego consciousness could also become, to differing degrees, dissociated from the more ancient affect-based substrata out of which it evolved. It was this dissociation that Jung believed gave rise not only to individual mental suffering, but also the malaise and suffering of social collectivities. Additionally, it was the integration of those two systems (what Jung referred to as individuation) that had become one of the most important tasks of human cultural development. For Jung, any future sane and healthy civilisation would be one that had become conscious of this dissociation and sought to heal it – not only at the individual but also collective level.

Jung and Early Anthropology: Bachofen and Australian Ethnography

In addition to Darwin and the paleoanthropological discoveries of the period, the late nineteenth and early twentieth centuries saw the rise of anthropology as a serious discipline. One of the major questions these early researchers were interested in was the nature of the archaic ancestors of modern humans. In much the same way as modern evolutionary anthropologists study contemporary hunter-gatherer societies in order to best understand Pleistocene hominins, nineteenth-century anthropologists also studied such cultures in their attempts to reconstruct the deep past.

The Pleistocene is the period from approximately 2 million years to 10,000 years ago. Humans were for the majority of this period hunter-gatherers. From 10,000 years to the present is the Holocene, the period that saw the emergence and global spread of agricultural societies with complex social stratification and economic hierarchies. This change in subsistence pattern is often referred as the Neolithic or agricultural revolution. It was during this period that agriculture, writing and specialist social classes such as scribes and a professional military class developed. During 10,000 and 3,000 years, a global transformation had occurred with many societies having shifted from hunting and gathering to a subsistence strategy based on agriculture (Stephens et al. 2019). One of Jung's interests was the nature of pre-literate human cultures during the early Neolithic and before the emergence of complex civilisations and writing, what he calls the 'old tribal doctrines that extended far back into Neolithic times and thus into a time of remarkable spiritual pregnancy and tension that dissolved only with the invention of the written word' (Jung and Neumann 2015: 59).

The *Homo erectus* and Neanderthal fossils Jung referred to in the above discussion were Pleistocene hominins. Given they were hunter-gatherers – as evidenced by archaeological deposits of hunting technologies found with the fossils – contemporary humans who share this subsistence pattern may assist in reconstructions of the deep past. This was essentially the approach of early anthropology. And Jung in his desire to understand the lifeways of our archaic ancestors who lived prior to the Neolithic revolution adopted this method.

Jung's life coincided with the growth of anthropology as a serious intellectual discipline. Importantly, it was around the time of his dream of descending the various stories of a house, to find in the lowest layer the skulls of fossil hominins, that Jung began seriously reading the anthropological literature and studies of mythology. This was research motivated by Jung's perception of the 'close relationship between ancient mythology' and the psychology of so-called 'primitive' cultures. It was also around this time that he turned to 'phylogeny to provide a basis for the understanding of individual development.' As Shamdasani elaborates, these 'psychobiological researches were linked to his anthropological reading: for the assumption of phylogenetic inheritance led to the view that the "data" on what was inherited would be provided by anthropology. Thus anthropology could provide a window into mankind's collective inheritance' (Shamdasani 2003: 295).

During this time, Jung synthesised human evolution and anthropology with what he learnt from comparative anatomy, developmental embryology and the putative relationship between ontogeny and phylogeny. In a sense, the various strands of his thinking began to converge – the biological theories that he inherited from the *Naturphilosophen*, palaeoanthropology and the nascent field of anthropology.

The anthropological paradigms which Jung would have encountered, particularly in the late nineteenth and early twentieth centuries, would have been predominantly in the evolutionary tradition, a tradition which sought to integrate ethnographic data with palaeoanthropology and archaeology in order to reconstruct the deep human past. Many twentieth-century assessments of that tradition, particularly in its second half and into the current century, have been if not all at least mostly negative. There are good reasons for this.

Most important among these is that many of Darwin's ideas, as well the surrounding cultural discourses, were underpinned by ethnocentric and racist conceptions of Indigenous people (Diogo 2024). Such views were also common elements in the anthropology of the period, which associated the ethnocentric ranking of races and putative measures of intelligence based on brain size, with the racist notion that Indigenous peoples were cognitively inferior to Europeans (Gould 1996). Such ideas played no small part in colonial attitudes towards Indigenous people, which served to justify colonial expansion, annexation of traditional lands and the cartographic enclosure of Indigenous ecological space (Ryan 1996; Carter 2013; McGregor 2015; Bhandar 2018).

However, this is only part of the story. While some of the attitudes of early anthropologists and those who studied Indigenous cultures are deemed ethically problematic by contemporary standards, those early researchers were often the most progressive members of *their* society. This is important to keep in my mind when judging their writings and the language they used by the moral standards of today (Morphy 1997). There is a paradox here: while early anthropology was influenced by the racist and ethnocentric attitudes of the culture of which it was a part, it also served to undermine that ethnocentrism by enabling the broader public to understand Indigenous cultures. This process had real world positive consequences, particularly when anthropologists became advocates for policy reform and the overturning of colonial and ethnocentric attitudes (Stanner and Manne 2011).

Emerging scholarship has also reassessed the merit of late nineteenth- and early twentieth-century traditions in anthropology. This reconsideration focusses on the importance of its evolutionary approach and analysis of kinship, religion, and sexual politics, which are in many ways consistent with modern ethnographic field data and which also serve to illuminate research issues in contemporary evolutionary theory (Knight 1995; Fox 1980, 2011; Chapais 2009; Power, Finnegan, and Callan 2017). As Chris Knight writes, in his defence of this tradition, for the early anthropologists 'Enlightenment was an end in itself; their own new science was an important aspect of the gradually advancing self-awareness of humankind' (Knight 1995: 63).

Important early theorists who shaped the general intellectual environment that impacted Jung's thought, or who had a direct influence on the development of analytical psychology throughout the twentieth century, include Johan Jacob Bachofen (1815–1887), Lewis Henry Morgan (1818–1881), Lucien Lévy-Bruhl (1857–1939), Emile Durkheim (1858–1917), Baldwin Spencer (1860–1929), Francis Gillen (1855–1912), Marcel Mauss (1872–1950), Henri Hubert (1872–1927) and Robert Briffault (1874–1948). One of the most influential approaches was the Bachofen-Morgan model which postulated the existence of an ancient form of matrilineal social organisation prior to the emergence of patriarchy. This paradigm signalled the emergence of modern kinship studies and the attempt to reconstruct the ancient evolutionary past of modern humans.

What was lacking however from the Bachofen-Morgan model was extensive ethnographic field data of extant hunter-gatherers. Some of the major clarifications came from field data collected by Baldwin Spencer (1860–1929) and Francis Gillen (1855–1912) who undertook research among the Aranda people, an Indigenous language group in Central Australia who live in the region surrounding the remote town of Alice Springs.

Spencer and Gillen's *The Native Tribes of Central Australia* (1899) and *The Northern Tribes of Central Australia* (1904) revolutionised anthropology. Mainly due to their association with Sir James Frazer and English Darwinists, the approach of Spencer and Gillen was evolutionary in its broad orientation (Spencer, Marett, and Penniman 1932). The impact that Spencer and Gillen's field work among the Aranda had on the trajectory of European intellectual history cannot be overstated. The popularity of their work and how it transformed the European conception of human culture and religion are often forgotten today. But that cultural amnesia, and the associated assumption that their work is predicted on colonial prejudice and therefore of little relevance to contemporary thought, has been subject to serious scholarly challenge in recent decades (Morphy 1988, 1997; Gillen et al. 1997).

At the time Spencer and Gillen's works were published, European researchers were engaged in complex debates about the nature of prehistory and the development of agriculture, city states and the emergence of complex civilisations. The nature of the social structures, religious practices and marriage systems that preceded these historical developments were debated intensely with the proliferation of speculative theories many of which lacked any empirical evidentiary basis. The works of Spencer and Gillen signalled a profound shift in how these questions were addressed. Their rigorous collection of data, their extensive cross checking among numerous informants, and their critical appraisal of theories developed by researchers in Europe, placed anthropology on a more solid empirical footing than had previously been the case.

Spencer and Gillen's ethnographies became key source texts for thinkers in Europe; most notable among them were Sir James Frazer (1854–1941) and Emile Durkheim (1858–1917) (Spencer, Marett, and Penniman 1932; Morphy 1988, 1997: 24–8). It could be argued that French sociology is an elaboration of Spencer and Gillen's ethnographic work, so important was it to the development of Durkheim's thought. For example, Durkheim used Spencer and Gillen's works as key texts in his 1912 *The Elementary Forms of Religious Life* as did Lévy-Bruhl in his 1935

Primitive Mythology: The Mythic World of the Australian and Papuan Natives.
Importantly, Lévy-Bruhl's text was one of Jung's main sources on Aboriginal Australians. Jung also frequently quotes directly from the works of Spencer and Gillen.
Importantly, Jung himself was explicit about the connection between his own ideas
and those of Marcel Mauss and Durkheim, arguing that his theory of archetypes
and the French sociological notion of 'categories' of the imagination are describing
the same phenomena (Jung 2014a: 79).

Scholars have noted the affinities – and differences – between the work of Jung
and Durkheim in their attempt to develop a 'depth sociology' (Greenwood 2013;
Goodwyn 2014). And Jung's use of Lévy-Bruhl's works is well known (Segal
2007). However, as I will suggest in the following discussion, many of the affinities between Jung's thought and French sociology seem to derive from the fact that
they were drawing on the same ethnographic source material – that is the field work
among the Aranda undertaken by Spencer and Gillen. More specifically, Durkheim
noted the connection between women's blood and the blood of the hunt, and how
blood came to symbolically represent the sacred dimension of life (Knight and
Lewis 2016: 87). Consequently, what are of particular significance for both Jung
and Durkheim are ochre (symbolic of blood), sacred stones or *churingas* (often
coated with ochre) and how these cultural objects are integral aspects of Indigenous ritual, kinship systems and the concept of the Dreaming. These aspects of
Jung's thought, and how they link his ideas to French sociology and Australian
ethnography, have yet to be explored in any detail by Jungian scholars – although
see Shamdasani for a brief discussion (Shamdasani 2003: 295–7).

Before looking at these issues in greater detail, I briefly discuss the Bachofen-
Morgan model which provides the context for anthropological debate in the nineteenth and early twentieth centuries.

Bachofen and Morgan: Analytical Psychology and Matrilineal Social Organisation

At the time Spencer and Gillen undertook their revolutionary research among the
Aranda, two of the most influential theorists in Europe were Johan Jacob Bachofen
(1815–1887) and Lewis Henry Morgan (1818–1881). Bachofen and Morgan laid
the foundations for modern kinship theory and postulated that a primitive form of
matrilineal social organisation preceded the emergence of the patriarchal nuclear
family. In many senses, they set the terms of debate for Australian ethnography
and provided abundant research questions that needed resolution. What Australian ethnography – and particularly the work of Spencer and Gillen – contributed
to debates in Europe was detailed and extensive field data. This had been largely
lacking up until this point. Importantly, Spencer and Gillen addressed many of the
questions raised by the Bachofen-Morgan model and were able to resolve a number of them. In this sense, they shifted anthropology out of the realm of specula-
tion into that of empirically based field work focussed on particular local cultures
(Morphy 1997: 25–7 and 42).

Bachofen published his *Mutterecht* in 1861, a work which was highly influential in stimulating debate about early forms of social organisation and the possibility of matrilineal forms of kinship in antiquity. Bachofen's theories were controversial at the time they were published as they 'shook the previously unchallenged notion that the patriarchal family' characterised the entirety of human history (Ellenberger 1970: 221). For example, Durkheim wrote in his 1912 *The Elementary Forms of Religious Life* that 'before the middle of the nineteenth century ... people were convinced that the father was the essential element of the family; a familial organization that did not hinge on the power of the father was inconceivable. Bachofen's discovery overturned this old idea' (Durkheim 2008: 8). And in his 1927 *The Mothers*, Robert Briffault praised Bachofen for perceiving 'one of the most momentous and fundamental facts of social history' going on to suggest that Bachofen stands in 'the highest place among the founders of modern social science' (Briffault 1927: 408–9).

Jung read Bachofen in his early years, which stimulated his interest in the Demeter myth, Dionysian ritual and the role of female symbolism in antiquity (Bair 2003: 33, 188 and footnote 662). While Jung rarely mentions Bachofen in his writings, there is additional evidence of the influence of Bachofen's matriarchal model on his thinking, particularly in letters he wrote to Freud in which he questioned the patriarchal assumptions of Freud's Oedipus theory (Ellenberger 1970: 223; Freud, Jung, and McGuire 1974: 502–3). The debate over an early stage of matrilineal social structure was one of the central points of contention in the early development of psychoanalysis, with Jung and figures like Otto Rank and Eric Fromm questioning the anthropological basis of Freud's theory (Clark 2020: 130–1). Reflecting on this debate, Burston avers that the 'continual conflict that in Freud's theory characterises the transition from our early hominid ancestors to civilisation was deferred by Bachofen to the later, warlike patriarchal period' (Burston 1991: 44).

Bachofen undertook extensive research of legal documents and artefacts from the ancient world concluding that female symbolism in antiquity was an expression of an early matrilineal social structure (Bachofen 1967: 144). Bachofen based this theory on the fact that the relationship between mother and child is the primary social bond, a bond that forms the foundation of social life more generally. As he writes:

> The relationship which stands at the origin of all culture, of every virtue, of every nobler aspect of existence, is that between mother and child; it operates in a world of violence as the divine principle of love, of union, of peace. Raising her young, the woman learns earlier than the man to extend her loving care beyond the limits of the ego to another creature, and to direct whatever gift of invention she possesses to the preservation and improvement of this other's existence. Woman at this stage is the repository of all culture, of all benevolence, of all devotion, of all concern for the living and grief for the dead.
>
> (Bachofen 1967: 79)

Bachofen's *Mutterecht* and Briffault's *The Mothers* became key texts in the development of analytical psychology in the twentieth century. These texts provided abundant evidence of female symbolism in antiquity and its putative relationship to social structure and religious life. Importantly, Briffault noted the widely reported association between cultural taboos, women's sexual function and lunar cycles. Briffault suggests, citing Darwin's research on the association between the mating cycles of marine creatures and lunar cycles, that such taboos may have an ancient evolutionary origin (Briffault 1927: 429).

In *Woman's Mysteries: Ancient and Modern*, Esther Harding built on Briffault's insights in her Jungian analysis of the association between menstruation and lunar cycles (Harding 1936: 57 and 92). Erich Neumann developed a similar approach in numerous works building on the work of both Bachofen and Briffault, most notably in *The Great Mother: An Analysis of the Archetype* and *The Fear of the Feminine and Other Essays on Feminine Psychology* (Neumann 1994, 2015). Significantly, this association between female reproductive cycles and the moon is a surprisingly recurrent cross-cultural motif, with women during their menstrual cycles being considered to be under the influence of the moon (Power 2022).

Lewis Henry Morgan provided further evidence for Bachofen's thesis in his *Systems of Consanguinity and Affinity of the Human Family* (1871) and *Ancient Society* (1877). In the latter, concurring with Bachofen, he argued that that the change of descent from the female to the male line negatively impacted women (Morgan 1985: 351). This resulted from women no longer residing in the communal household of their matrilineal kin group, but residing with their husband, which eventually laid the foundation of the monogamous family unit. When residing with matrilineal kin, women can utilise those kin-based alliances if conflict arises with other individuals. Such support is lost, in Morgan's view, if she resides with the husband or her husband's family (Morgan 1985: 350–1).

Morgan had found affinities between Bachofen's analysis of documents, myth and art in classical antiquity and the social organisation of the Iroquois, a Native American people whose kinship structure he had studied. So compelling was the case made by Bachofen and Morgan that at the turn of the twentieth century, virtually 'all those who had helped found the discipline of anthropology converged around the fundamentals of the Bachofen-Morgan theory' (Knight 2009: 69). During Jung's formative years and well into the twentieth century, this was a widely accepted model of human historical development and one of the assumed premises of the anthropological thought of the period. However, by the mid-twentieth century, this paradigm had been all but abandoned, in part due to shortcomings of the theory itself, but more as a result of political and sociocultural factors (Knight 2009). Only in recent years has the Bachofen-Morgan model been reappraised based on confirmatory evidence from contemporary anthropological field work.

The rejection of nineteenth- and early twentieth-century anthropology, and the evolutionary approach to human development that grew out of the Western Enlightenment, had a significant impact on Jungian scholarship. The consequence was that many Jungians, understandably, seemed to be wary and sceptical about early anthropological models due to their frequent association with racist and colonial ideologies – ideologies that are at times not only implicit but also explicit in some aspects of Jung's thought (Dalal 1988; Samuels 2019). However, this is only part of the story, and while early anthropology gave expression to, and was often used to buttress, racist ideologies, it was much more than this. Current scholarly reassessment of this tradition makes this abundantly clear. In what follows, I explore Jung's thought in light of that reassessment.

Jung and the Dreaming: Spencer and Gillen and Indigenous Ontology

One of the central aspects of classical Aboriginal Australian culture is the notion of the Dreaming. The Dreaming is not only the creative period during which ancestral beings traversed the landscape and created its specific geological features and flora and fauna. It is also active in the present and becomes manifest in ritual and dreamlife. In this sense, it constitutes a parallel reality, one full of sacred significance that exists side by side with profane existence. However, the membrane separating these two domains is permeable and can be passed through during ritual and dreamlife.

The concept of the Dreaming, along with many other aspects of Aranda culture, was first fully explicated and explained to a European readership by Spencer and Gillen in *The Native Tribes of Central Australia*. As anthropologist Howard Morphy writes:

> The significance of their work lies in their analysis which set the framework for future research in Australia, and which presented data on Aboriginal societies in such a way that it transformed previous understandings of them. The key concepts and themes that subsequently became associated with Aboriginal religion – the network of ancestral tracks that intersect the landscape, the distribution of rights in sacred knowledge, the locality-based nature of much ritual practice, the complex relationship between totemism (or sacred knowledge) and social groups and, perhaps the most significant of all, the Dreamtime – were all established in Spencer and Gillen's writings. Their work produced an immensely more complex view of Aboriginal religion than had existed before – a view that has lasted both as ethnography and as an agenda that influenced subsequent research.
>
> (Morphy 1997: 37)

Spencer and Gillen based the concept of the Dreamtime on the Aranda word *alcheringa*. The notion of the Dreamtime, as a specific time in the past, has been rejected by contemporary researchers. The most currently used translation is the Dreaming – which does not specify a time in the past but recognises the atemporal nature of the Dreaming (Hume 2002: 24–37). That is, the Dreaming exists just as much in the past as it does in the present and future – in fact to frame it in terms of past, present and future is probably to misunderstand the atemporal nature of the Dreaming. Nevertheless, Spencer and Gillen's elaboration on this concept, and its relationship with other aspects of Aranda social and religious life was a major contribution to Western understanding of Indigenous Australian culture. Their detailed ethnography enabled other Australians and the broader international community to better understand Indigenous cultures – a process that continues to this day.

More recent analyses have highlighted specific cultural articulations of this concept among different Indigenous language groups in Australia. For example, among the Walpiri people the Dreaming and the potency of such ancestral power (*djugurba* in Walpiri) is thought to be hidden from everyday view, that is 'split off' from the sensory field of waking consciousness, only to be made manifest in dream and ritual (Munn 1973: 103). Similarly, Pintupi ontology frames existence in terms of a 'split cosmos' – for example, *yuti* means something which is seen or visible, whereas as *tjukurrpa*, which translates as 'dreaming,' usually connotes something which is hidden and, as with the Walpiri concept, made manifest in dream or in ritual (Myers 1991: 48–9 and 243).

The concept of the Dreaming is an important aspect of Jung's writings on religion, ritual and scared objects. For example, in *Psychology and Alchemy*, Jung states that 'ancestral spirits play an important part in primitive rites of renewal' going on to state that 'the aborigines of central Australia even identify themselves with their mythical ancestors of the *alcheringa* period, a sort of Homeric age' (Jung 1980: 131). He also states that for 'primitive' or Indigenous cultures, the 'mythical world of [the] ancestors - for instance, the *alchera* or *bugari* of the Australian aborigines - is a reality equal if not superior to the material world.' Jung does not provide any citation here but in a footnote writes that this 'fact is well known, and the relevant ethnological literature is too extensive to be mentioned here' (Jung 2014a: 154). It is likely that Jung's specific source for this quote was from *Primitive Mythology* where Lévy-Bruhl writes that in 'Australian and New Guinea tribes words like *altjira, dzjugur, bugari* … combine the connotations of "dream experience" and "the mythic period and all that it involves"' (Lévy-Bruhl 1983: 16).

Jung used Australian ethnography to infer possible functions of ritual during the Stone Age – which is another way of describing the pre-Neolithic or preagricultural period in human historical development. Jung suggested that the performance of sacred rituals has a beneficent social and psychological function and that the need for group identification that such rituals cultivate is a very ancient human impulse structured into evolutionarily ancient layers of the brain. As he writes emphasising the importance of such rituals for social life:

> … the Australian conception of the *alcheringamijina* … ancestral souls, half man and half animal, whose reactivation through religious rites is of the greatest functional significance for the life of the tribe. Ideas of this sort, dating back to the Stone Age, were widely diffused, as may be seen from numerous other traces that can be found elsewhere.
>
> (Jung 2014a: 125)

Jung's emphasis on the social role of such rites – that is their 'functional signifi-cance for the life of the tribe' – indicates that far from focussing merely on psychol-ogy, and avoiding social structure, Jung was in many ways adopting a sociological conception of the psyche. Importantly, such identification with the group is coupled with identification with ancestral beings, which Jung associates with evolutionar-ily ancient brain systems. This, he argues, is most likely a characteristic of human cultures during the Stone Age – that is cultures prior to the invention of metal-based technologies: as he writes 'the regressive identification with lower and more primitive states of consciousness is invariably accompanied by a heightened sense of life; hence the quickening effect of regressive identifications with half-animal ancestors in the Stone Age' (Jung 2014a: 125). Jung cites both Lévy-Bruhl's *Primi-tive Mythology* and Spencer and Gillen's *The Northern Tribes of Central Australia* as his source on these issues. As already noted, Spencer and Gillen were two of the main sources Lévy-Bruhl used in *Primitive Mythology*. What similarities ex-ist between Jung's ideas and Lévy-Bruhl's – as well as French sociology more generally – owe much to their reliance on the same ethnographic source material.

Jung argues that such rites are a form of psychotherapy that facilitate the inte-gration of the unconscious with consciousness – that is a form of individuation. However, given the fraught nature of the emergence of consciousness out of the unconscious, and the potential dangers involved in the process of integration, indi-viduation needs to be managed thoughtfully and sensitively. These dangers include the potential for insanity, psychosis and dissociative disorders. In this sense, such rites are designed to facilitate the healthy integration of the unconscious and to mitigate any potential dangers. As he writes:

> Because man has consciousness, a development of this kind [individuation] does not run very smoothly; often it is varied and disturbed, because consciousness deviates again and again from its archetypal, instinctual foundation and finds it-self in opposition to it. There then arises the need for a synthesis of the two posi-tions. This amounts to psychotherapy even on the primitive level, where it takes the form of restitution ceremonies. As examples I would mention the identifica-tion of the Australian aborigines with their ancestors in the *alcheringa* period.
> (Jung 2014a: 39–40)

Jungian scholars to date have only provided a cursory analysis of Jung's indebt-edness to Spencer and Gillen (Dalal 1988: 3; Petchkovsky, Roque, and Beskow 2003: 215–6; Shamdasani 2003: 292; Tacey 2009: 28–9; Samuels 2019: 219). A number of these discussions claim that the works of Spencer and Gillen informed Jung's racism. For example, in his discussion in *Psychological Types* (Jung 1991: 30) of Indigenous people not differentiating between subjective experiences and objective reality to the degree Europeans do, Jung quotes Spencer and Gillen. In the passage – which both Dalal and Samuels quote as evidence of Jung's racism – Spencer and Gillen write that what 'a savage experiences during a dream is just as real to him as what he sees when he is awake' (Dalal 1988: 3; Samuels 2019: 219).

Obviously, the use of the term savage tends not to be acceptable to modern sensibilities due to its negative associations. It should be noted, however, that it was a common term of the period and continued to be used in France well into the twentieth century – for example, in Levi Strauss' classic *The Savage Mind* which was first published in French in 1962. Consequently, the term may not have had for Spencer and Gillen all of the negative connotations it does for modern readers.

While many of the quotations Dalal and Samuels cite in their articles do provide evidence of Jung's racism, it is debatable whether the passage from Spencer and Gillen which Jung cites can be counted among such evidence. In order to give the broader context of this comment – which Samuels admits to not providing – I will quote the passage in full from Spencer and Gillen's *The Native Tribes of Central Australia*. It is important to note that Spencer and Gillen are referring to a crucial aspect of Indigenous ontology in which the notion of distinct essences is seemingly obviated. During ritual transformations of consciousness, humans, sacred objects, ancestral beings and the totemic geography of the landscape, are considered to be manifestations of the same essence – that is the Dreaming. Humans maintain a link to that domain of existence through ritual life and dream. When discussing the relationship between dreamlife, ritual and *iruntarinia* or spirit individuals, Spencer and Gillen write:

> What a savage experiences during a dream is just as real to him as what he sees when he is awake. The natives have a very definite conception of the spirit part of an individual, and imagine that during sleep it can and does wander about freely. Their thoughts at certain times are so much occupied with the performance of sacred ceremonies that very naturally the latter enter into their dreams, with the result that the more highly imaginative ones believe that they have actually been in the company of the *iruntarinia*, and that the latter have shown them the ceremonies which in reality they invent, based probably upon the recollection of what they have seen during a dream.
>
> (Spencer and Gillen 1904: 451)

In their discussion of this aspect of Indigenous religious phenomenology, Spencer and Gillen highlight that it is only a select few individuals who are capable of interacting with *iruntarinia* in this manner and their ability to do so is highly valued by the rest of the community. As they write, there are 'special individuals who are supposed to have the power of seeing the spirits' who 'every now and then show them sacred ceremonies.' They continue adding that it 'is only a very few men amongst the Arunta and Kaitish tribes who thus claim to and are regarded by their fellows as able to see and hold intercourse with the *iruntarinia*' (Spencer and Gillen 1904: 450 and 51).

Importantly, it is through interactions with the *iruntarinia* that these individuals become medicine men or healers – or as the anthropologist A.P. Elkin called them in the book of that name Aboriginal men of high degree (Elkin 1993). As I will elaborate in Chapter 5, in his classic cross-cultural study of shamanism, Mircea

Eliade used Elkin as his source for Australia, noting the similarities between our local medicine men or healers and shamanic practices across the globe. One of the most salient similarities emerging from Eliade's cross-cultural study was the cultivation of visionary or altered states of consciousness and encounters with spirit entities – which Elkin noted was a central aspect of Aboriginal Australian traditions.

Spencer and Gillen allude to this phenomenon mentioning the making of a medicine man in which he has his internal organs removed and replaced by 'atnongara stones.' These stones, as they write, are 'small crystalline structures' which every medicine man is supposed to be able to 'produce at will from his body.' It is the possession of these stones which confers 'virtue to the medicine man' (Spencer and Gillen 1904: 480). However, it is likely that many of the accounts of being surgically operated on, having internal organs removed and replaced with crystals or magic stones – which are often recounted by informants in a realistic manner as if they happened in the material world – are most likely accounts of visionary states induced through ritual processes (Elkin 1993: 112).

These vivid accounts, which informants assure anthropologists really occurred, most likely acquire their powerful sense of verisimilitude due to the profoundly transformative nature of the experience. That is, not only are they real – they are often considered more real, and more important, than ordinary modes of waking consciousness. In fact, it would be inaccurate to say that such experiences are *not* real. They are aspects of our evolved neurophenomenology, and they have a profound sacred meaning to those who experience them. In every sense, they are veridical. As Jackson Lincoln states in his cross-cultural ethnography of dreaming, while Indigenous people do distinguish between dream and waking reality, 'dream experience' is thought to have 'greater reality value than an actual experience' (Lincoln 1970: 28). The same could be said of ritually induced alteration of consciousness, which seem to be subserved by the same neurobiological mechanisms as dreams (Hobson 2002, 2009; Carhart-Harris and Friston 2010; Hobson, Hong, and Friston 2014).

The essential point made by Spencer and Gillen is supported by modern ethnographic field work. Australian Indigenous religion is an example of a polyphasic culture that values other modes of consciousness in addition to normal waking consciousness – in fact often values them more. Those that live in monophasic cultures, with a predominantly rationalist orientation, are likely to find the sense of verisimilitude that Indigenous people attribute to dreamlife an alien and possibly incomprehensible conception of reality (Laughlin 2011: 62–6). The passage from Spencer and Gillen quoted above, and Jung's comment upon it, accurately reflects Indigenous Australian religious phenomenology and conceptions of ontology.

Sacred Stones: From Churingas to Alchemy

Churingas have a crucial role in Indigenous Australian religion. Churingas may be either sacred stones or wooden boards. Like body designs or sand mosaics used in ritual, they represent the ancestral beings associated with the creation of human beings as well as local flora, fauna and features of the landscape. Spencer and Gillen's work was responsible for elucidating the role *churingas* played in ritual life and kinship structures, and how the designs painted or engraved on them symbolised the journey of ancestral beings across vast tracts of country and their present embodiment in various features of the landscape. In this sense, such objects mediate the connection between the everyday reality of waking consciousness and the parallel or alternate reality of the Dreaming. It was because of their role as embodiments of ancestral power that *churingas* were often hidden away in caves away from women and the uninitiated only to be brought out of their sacred hiding places on ceremonial occasions.

One of the most important components of Jung's theory of symbolism is what he calls the 'dynamic relation between man and objects' (Jung 2014c). Jung has in mind here not just any objects but those which take on a sacred character and which are invested with numinous qualities. The crystalline 'atnongara stones' that medicine men acquire discussed above are Australian examples (Spencer and Gillen 1904: 480). In *Alchemical Studies*, Jung explores cross-cultural stone and gem symbolism from Western traditions such as the *lapis philosophorum* or philosopher's stone, to Native American and Australian examples (Jung 1953). A crucial component in Jung's theory, which enabled him to connect alchemy with the cross-cultural symbolism of sacred objects, came from his reading of Spenser and Gillen's analysis of Indigenous *churingas*.

When discussing sacred objects, Jung states that the '*churinga* of the Australian aborigine' represents a 'similar concept' to those found cross-culturally. For Jung, the *churingas* are 'ritual objects' that represent 'the body of an individual ancestor (from whom the life force comes)' – noting that the concept can be extended to 'the mystical property of any object' (Jung 2014c: 90). This is generally correct – while *churingas* are most commonly known in the form of stones or boards with sacred designs on them, any object with such designs can potentially be referred to as *churinga* – for example, such designs on features of the landscape such as rock shelters or cave walls. The passage Jung is referring to, and which he quotes in the footnote comes from Spencer and Gillen's *The Northern Tribes of Central Australia*. I quote the passage in full from the original text, which is accompanied by a photograph of a *churinga* with a snake design on it:

> The native has a vague and undefined but still a very strong idea that any sacred object such as a Churinga, which has been handed down from generation to generation, is not only endowed with the magic power put into it when first it was made, but has gained some kind of virtue from every individual to whom it has belonged. A man who owns such a Churinga as this snake one will constantly rub it over with his hand, singing as he does so the Alcheringa history of the snake, and gradually comes to feel that there is some special association between him and the sacred object—that a virtue of some kind passes from it to him and also from him to it.
>
> (Spencer and Gillen 1904: 277)

In his *Alchemical Studies*, Jung develops these ideas in the context of a discussion of stone symbolism:

> The stone as the birth place of the gods (e.g., the birth of Mithras from a stone) is attested by primitive legends of stone births which go back to ideas that are even more ancient—for instance, the view of the Australian aborigines that children's souls live in a special stone called the "child-stone." They can be made to migrate into a uterus by rubbing the "child-stone" with a *churinga. Churingas* may be boulders, or oblong stones artificially shaped and decorated, or oblong, flattened pieces of wood ornamented in the same way. They are used as cult instruments. The Australians and the Melanesians maintain that *churingas* come from the totem ancestor, that they are relics of his body or of his activity, and are full of *arunquiltha* or mana. They are united with the ancestor's soul and with the spirits of all those who afterwards possess them. They are taboo, are buried in caches or hidden in clefts in the rocks. In order to "charge" them, they are buried among the graves so that they can soak up the mana of the dead. They promote the growth of field produce, increase the fertility of men and animals, heal wounds, and cure sicknesses of the body and the soul ... The *churingas* used for ceremonial purposes are daubed with red ochre, anointed with fat, bedded or wrapped in leaves, and copiously spat on (spittle = mana).
>
> (Jung 1953: 97)

One of the crucial things mentioned here is the fact that churingas are often painted with ochre. In Indigenous Australian religions, ochre symbolises blood which is itself considered to be scared. As already noted, blood also has important associations with menstruation, the blood of animals and ritual life – as I explore in more detail in Chapters 3 and 5. Importantly, as highlighted by Spencer and Gillen, there is a link between mythology and the symbolic ritualised use of ochre. For example, Aboriginal myths explaining the origin of ochre deposits in Australia often associate them with female fertility. Spencer and Gillen comment upon such associations in their *The Native Tribes of Central Australia*. For instance, during the creation period, female ancestral beings created ochre deposits with their sexual organs while dancing. As already noted, *churingas* are often covered with such ochre deposits (Spencer and Gillen 2000: 442 and 568).

Paraphrasing the observations of Spencer and Gillen regarding ochre and mythology, Durkheim writes in *The Elementary Forms of Religious Life*:

> First of all, human blood is so holy that the tribes of central Australia very often use it to consecrate the most respected cultic instruments. In certain cases the *nurtunja* [a vertical pole-like structure used in ritual] for example, is religiously anointed from top to bottom with human blood. Among the Arunta, men of the Emu clan draw the sacred emblem on ground completely soaked in blood. [...] Moreover, the religious nature of blood also explains the religious role of red ochre and its frequent use in certain ceremonies; the *churingas* are rubbed with

it, and it is used in ritual decorations. Red ochre is thought to be a substance related to blood because of its colour. Several deposits of red ochre found at different sites on Arunta territory are said to be coagulated blood that certain heroines of the mythic period had shed on the ground.

(Durkheim 2008: 106)

Note that Jung referred to *churingas* as 'cult instruments' as does Durkheim – additionally, both note the association with blood and these sacred objects. The shared source for this association is Spencer and Gillen. Significantly, excavations from a 40,000-year-old burial site in Willandra Lakes in New South Wales in Australia revealed an individual who was buried covered in ochre (Bowler et al. 2003). This provides the suggestion that ochre and its symbolic associations may be of great antiquity and may have been part of the cultural complex Indigenous people's brought with them as they migrated through South East Asia and into Australia tens of thousands of years ago. Such antiquity is suggested by evidence of ochre and possible ritualised use as early as 500,000 years ago in Africa (Watts, Chazan, and Wilkins 2016). This would mean that the symbolic use of ochre is extremely ancient and may have formed part of a source cosmology shared by all early human populations (Power 2017).

Numerous scholars have sought to formulate a *depth sociology* by synthesising depth psychology and sociology. The possibility of such a synthesis is feasible, according to these authors, because there exists already significant affinities between the work of Jung and Durkheim (Staude 1976; Greenwood 2013; Goodwyn 2014). However, as well as similarities, these authors also point out significant differences between Jung and Durkheim. Staude has argued that Jung was 'on the road away from narrow individualistic and reductive positivism towards a *social* theory of culture and consciousness.' That is, there is an existent, yet incipient and yet to be fully formed sociology of the psyche in Jung's writings. Consequently, he argues that despite their similarities, Jung 'never quite realized how society can carry the moral order, as Durkheim did.' Staude argues that when Jung spoke of the collective unconscious he meant the 'collective, transpersonal dimension in the individual psyche.' The implication for Staude is that this diminishes the sociological significance of Jung's approach. The other theoretical impasse that prevented Jung from developing a fully formed sociology, according to Staude, was that 'he never fully succeeded in extricating himself from his original biological and energy models' (Staude 1976: 316).

It is not clear why Jung's biological approach precludes the development of a nuanced sociological approach in analytical psychology. In the context of the evolutionary and sociological approaches explored in this book, far from being mutually exclusive, sociology and evolutionary biology seem to be eminently compatible. However, this requires a slight change of emphasis from how sociological approaches to culture and biological theories of the mind have historically been conceived. Biology does not preclude culture; in fact, it seems that culture is the expression of our evolved biology. For example, human kinship systems and the formation of moral communities and the attendant symbols and rituals, seem to be in large part a result of evolutionary process. They are the objective expressions of the unique anatomy, neurobiology and trajectories of brain and somatic development characteristic of the human species. As Fox notes, the 'categories of mind may well be social in origin, but this is a true phylogenetic origin and not a culturally learned ontogenetic origin. Thus we carry society within our minds, as Durkheim saw, but not simply because we incorporate it through socialization: It is in us to start with' (Fox 1980: 192).

When we analyse the approaches of Jung and Durkheim to ritual and social life, particularly when focussing on ochre and sacred objects, similarities between the two thinkers become more salient. For example, while Jung focusses on the psychological his ideas about the historical development of consciousness are actually part of a broader sociological analysis. For example, his analysis of the historical development of ancient kinship structures, and their cultural and symbolic elaboration in alchemy, is by his own admission 'sociological' (Jung 1983: 63). Importantly, one of his main sources in that analysis of the historical transformation of social and kinship structures is Spencer Gillen (Jung 1983: 66). Additionally, Jung's conception of libido was one grounded in an analysis of the evolution of social structure; as he writes commenting on 'kinship' libido:'[i]ncest, as an endogamous relationship, is an expression of the libido which serves to hold the family together' (Jung 1983: 62). Additionally, religious rituals did not evolve as individual but as social activities; as he avers, religious rites have 'the greatest functional significance for the life of the tribe' (Jung 2014a: 125).

While Jung, the psychologist, placed importance on sociological analysis, Durkheim the sociologist, placed significant importance on psychological factors. For example, Durkheim writes that social life is 'entirely psychic, made up exclusively of objectified ideas and feelings,' that 'religious life cannot reach a certain degree of intensity without involving a psychic exaltation that is in some way akin to delirium' and that what 'makes a thing holy is ... the collective feeling attached to it' (Durkheim 2008: 271 and 308). He also emphasises the role of ritual in stimulating ecstatic emotional states, even connecting ritual with prophecy, psychoactive liquor, visions and what today we would refer to as altered states of consciousness (Durkheim 2008: 171–2 and 304). In addition to shared concerns about the symbolism of blood, sacred objects and kinship, the above discussion suggests quite salient affinities between Jung the psychologist and Durkheim the sociologist.

An important point to emphasise here is that while Durkheim was able to elucidate the relationship between taboos, sacred objects, the identification of women's blood with the blood of the hunt, he was according to Knight and Lewis unable to provide an explanation as to why these associations existed (Knight and Lewis 2016: 89). Nevertheless, Durkheim did an outstanding job of assembling the various pieces together. As Knight writes when commenting on the Aboriginal belief that a 'man might really be a kangaroo,' Durkheim did not reject the notion as ir-rational, but saw it as a manifestation of the mind's metaphorical capacity. As he writes with 'extraordinary insight' Durkheim

> ... realized that communal activities of this metaphorical kind lie at the basis of all symbolic thinking ... In Durkheim's evolutionary narrative, totemism and ex-ogamy emerge together as the earliest form of ritual and social organization. Com-munal participation in dancing, singing and other ritual performance forges bonds of solidarity while, at the same time, body and mind are seized by a metaphorical representation of their existence as a collective. That metaphor – the 'totem' – is the creature whose movements and appearance are acted out in the dance.
>
> (Knight and Lewis 2016: 87)

It is such metaphorical representations Jung was referring to when he wrote of the 'identification of the Australian aborigines with their ancestors in the *alcheringa* period (Jung 2014a: 39–40). Durkheim also noted how the association between women's blood and the blood of the hunt served an important social function. As Knight writes, women 'repulse the other sex with their symbolically potent blood' with women's blood also being equated with the blood of 'a kangaroo or other game animal.' The result is that certain women establish themselves as 'sacred beings' and consequently 'sexually prohibited, just as meat of the totemic species becomes prohibited flesh' (Knight and Lewis 2016: 87). In this way, a 'powerful communal metaphor enforces a unitary principle of exogamy which applies alike to human and nonhuman kin' (Knight and Lewis 2016: 87 and 88). Despite these key insights however, Knight argues that Durkheim's theory fails to explain crucial issues. As he avers:

> Durkheim offers no simple, logical explanation for its key feature – the iden-tification of women's blood with the blood of the hunt. Durkheim marshals ethnographic details confirming that across Australia, blood does have this sym-bolic significance, but he does not explain how or why hunter-gatherers across Australia should ever have arrived at that idea.
>
> (Knight and Lewis 2016: 86)

In his 1995 book *Blood Relations: Menstruation and the Origins of Culture* and consequent publications, Knight sought to answer these questions (Knight 1988, 1995, 2005, 2009; Knight and Power 2005; Knight and Lewis 2016). Knight outlined a theory of human evolution based on the cyclicity of female menstrual cycles. The existence of taboos around hunting and menstruation in foraging cultures, Knight argued, may have emerged in our evolutionary past as female coalitions sought to temper and redirect male violence – which with the advent of tools and weaponry during the Pleistocene could have posed quite a serious threat to social cohesion.

Importantly, hunting and menstruation both involve blood, which is linked to the sacred realm of life. If groups of women could collectively establish boundaries, and control male sexual and hunting behaviour, by redirecting it into socially pro-ductive avenues, this could have signalled the emergence of human culture and the origins of group level sociality and co-operation. If males adopted provisioning of their wives and own offspring as a reproductive strategy, this could enhance male reproductive success. The result would be hunting effort directed towards social cooperation in which males respect female solidarity and bring back game to the camp to share (Knight and Lewis 2016: 95). It is through this process that the blood of the hunt and female reproductive cycles and sexuality, became linked, giving rise to cross-cultural conceptions of the sacredness of blood and the associated ta-boos and prohibitions (Power, Sommer, and Watts 2013; Watts 2017; Power 2022).

The project of developing a *depth sociology* advocated by Jungians can be greatly enhanced by attending to the important role of blood symbolism, sacred objects and ritual in the work of both Jung and Durkheim. Their shared reliance on Spencer and Gillen highlights affinities that remain largely unexplored by Jungian scholars – lacunae in the extant analytical psychology literature the above discussion seeks to fill. The above analysis also hints at how an *evolutionary depth sociology* may be developed by exploring further intersections between Jung's thought and the model developed by Knight and colleagues – intersections I have explored elsewhere (Clark 2020). These issues will be discussed in more detail in Chapters 3 and 5.

The Reassessment of Evolutionary Stage Theory and Analytical Psychology

One of the major arguments of this book is that the traditions that formed Jung's evolutionary thinking, in terms of both developmental biology and anthropology, were effectively rejected by major currents in twentieth-century scientific thought. Jungian scholars followed these paradigmatic trends and as a consequence they often rejected Jung's evolutionary thinking, assuming its fundamental assumptions were invalid. However, this is no longer the case. In Chapter 1, I discussed how sci-entists have reassessed the *Naturphilosophen* and hence given renewed relevance to German comparative anatomy and developmental embryology and by implica-tion Jung's evolutionary thinking.

The anthropological traditions that Jung based his evolutionary ideas on have also been re-reassessed in recent years, after almost a century of being rejected as outdated and not worthy of serious consideration. In what follows, I discuss the reasons for the decline and rebirth of the anthropological traditions that Jung's ideas developed out of. Combined with the reassessment of the developmental tra-ditions in German biology that influenced Jung's thinking there is increased scope for analytical psychology to become aligned with – and to influence – some of the major trends in modern scientific thought.

The Enlightenment project that motivated nineteenth- and early twentieth-century anthropology, that is Morgan's mandate 'to explore the Universal History of Mankind' (Fox 2011: 318) became an intellectual causality of a number socio-cultural factors during the twentieth century. Quite legitimately, the association of such ideas with broader trends in the culture that buttressed colonial and racist ideologies led many to turn away from evolutionary approaches based on a putatively universal human nature. This resulted in increased focus on local cultural specificity, particularity, and difference. Additionally, the Bachofen-Morgan model was promoted by Marxists, which led to the rejection of such an approach for completely different reasons. Paradoxical as it may sound, the approach of Bachofen and Morgan was rejected for being associated with both colonial racism and Marxist communism.

One of the assumptions of early anthropology was that Indigenous people were primitive relics of a Stone Age or Palaeolithic culture. While it is most likely true that contemporary Indigenous cultures are more different to modern agricultural and industrial cultures than they are to humans living prior to the Neolithic revolution, they are not static relics of the deep past. This was one of the important observations made by Spencer and Gillen who recorded Aboriginal cultures themselves undergoing processes of transformation in the late nineteenth century (Morphy 1997: 33). However, the notion that they were a static relic of an earlier stage of evolution did often underpin the ethnocentric ranking of races characteristic of the period (Johnson and Earle 2022: 2–3; Way 2022). This conception also informed the evolutionary ranking of races according to putative correlations between intelligence and brain size – a view in which Africans and Australian Aboriginals were thought to occupy an inferior and lower rung of the evolutionary ladder (Gould 1996). Such evolutionary conceptions of race also informed colonial policy and the notion that races on a lower evolutionary rung were destined to die out and be replaced by more advanced races – the so-called 'doomed race' theory (McGregor 2015). The ethnocentric biases associated with such thinking are definitely evident in Jung's writings (Dalal 1988; Clark 2021: 5). However, I will argue that such approaches, purged of the ethnocentrism they were often imbued with, still have current utility. In fact, they are a crucial component in our contemporary understanding of human evolution, psychology and culture providing foundational insights relevant to current studies in evolutionary anthropology and the development of kinship systems.

Fox has attributed the decline and rejection of the universalist approach in anthropology to post-1968 cultural developments and the emergence of post-structuralism in the academy (Fox 2011: 315 and 17). This seems to be an important factor given post-structuralism and the development of postmodern perspectives in the works of Foucault and Derrida, for example, focussed on the language and cultural systems of European modernity. More specifically, they sought to critique the various means by which psychiatry, the biological sciences and anthropology were implicated in Western systems of discourse and power relations (Foucault 2005, 2013; Derrida 2016), an approach that was extended in Said's influential analysis of colonial representations of the colonised (Said 1995). While these were legitimate developments that highlighted the cultural embeddedness and contingencies of many aspects of European modernity and Enlightenment rationalism, the focus on cultural systems of representation effectively precludes from the outset any unequivocal empirical statements about the nature of reality.

The logical extension of such theories is a form of extreme idealism whereby culturally contingent representations are argued to be forever and inevitably divorced from the external world. This can lead to a position of epistemological nihilism where any recourse to empirical investigation of reality is interpreted as only ever a culturally contingent representation. From this perspective, all we can know is how the world is represented by cultural and ideological systems – representations that while revealing nothing about reality do reveal, when deconstructed, their own implicit ideological biases. Such critique formed the basis of post-structuralist and postmodern orientations in recent Jungian scholarship, particularly in relation to the influence of the biological sciences and Enlightenment knowledge systems on Jung's thought (Hauke 2000; Rowland 2002: 144; Rowland 2004; Gardner and Gray 2016).

Fox has argued that, as a result of these developments, universalist conceptions of the evolutionary emergence of humankind – that is, all humans as a species – were rejected by the anthropological profession. Consequently, anthropology tended to focus on the particularity of specific cultures while abandoning any attempt to understand how these cultures may be part of a larger more expansive conception of humankind. This entails failing to integrate particular field studies with research in other domains of knowledge such as palaeoanthropology, archaeology and the historical emergence of complex and hierarchised state-based societies from a more ancient hunter-gatherer subsistence pattern. As Fox writes of Morgan's historical stage model:

> The stages were like a ladder leading up vertically from the past. We simply took the ladder and moved it to the horizontal. It no longer led from anywhere to anywhere. We were left staring at all these rungs. What to do with them? We had acquired them because they were a ladder, and this ladder had given them an order and a meaning. But now they were simply there. The rungs were no longer related chronologically and causally to each other; each was just a different example of "cultural construction" in an unwinding and inexplicable diversity of cultural schemes. And none of them was connected to the biological processes of evolution in which the vertical ladder had logically placed them, its bottom rungs plunging into the evolutionary past.
>
> (Fox 2011: 318)

Another important factor leading to the demise of the Bachofen-Morgan model was political. Both Marx and Engels read Morgan's *Ancient Society* (1877) and were glad to have putative anthropological evidence of primitive communism and the possible existence of a stage of matrilineal social organisation prior to the emergence of the patriarchal nuclear family. Engels elaborated on Morgan's ideas and their implications for a materialist conception of history in his 1884 *The Origin of the Family, Private Property and the State* (Engels 2010). Engel's book popularised

Morgan's theories about human kinship, and during the ensuing years, Morgan's ideas became associated with communism – an association that played a crucial role in their demise among Western intellectuals, academics and anthropologists (Knight 2009; 1995: 61–2). As Robert Lowie wrote in his history of ethnographic theory, Morgan's *Ancient Society* '… attracted the notice of Marx and Engels, who accepted and popularized its evolutionary doctrines as being in harmony with their own philosophy.' Consequently, Morgan's book was translated into numerous European languages with the result that 'German workingmen would sometimes reveal an uncanny familiarity with the Hawaiian and Iroquois mode of designating kin, matters not obviously connected with a proletarian revolution' (Lowie 1987: 54).

The result of the association with Marxism was that the Bachofen-Morgan conception of human historical development effectively became an intellectual casualty of the Cold War. Reflecting on these issues, Marvin Harris has argued that the development of cultural anthropology in the twentieth century developed in reaction to Marxism; as he writes with 'Morgan's scheme incorporated into Communist doctrine, the struggling science of anthropology crossed the threshold of the twentieth century with a clear mandate for its own survival and well-being: expose Morgan's scheme and destroy the method on which it was based.' The consequence, according to Harris, is that anthropology abandoned the comparative method, as well as the attempt to view history from a nomothetic standpoint that could investigate generalised patterns (Harris 1968: 249).

Knight has commented on the two main avenues of attack against the Bachofen-Morgan model by anthropologists in the twentieth century. Those who were influenced by Franz Boas (1858–1942) rejected universalist conceptions of culture and the racist implications of 'Grand Theory' in favour of detailed description of specific cultures. However, they also had a specific political agenda. As Knight writes:

> On the one hand, they attacked racist and biological-reductionist theories of evolution and history; on the other, they aimed to demolish key Marxist notions such as that of 'primitive communism', arguing repeatedly – in direct opposition to Engels – that private property, the state and 'the family' were timeless universals of all human existence.
>
> (Knight 1995: 62)

The rejection of nineteenth-century anthropology represents a case study in ideology impacting the direction of science, giving some credence to the postmodern critique that science is part of, and deeply embedded in, broader ideological and cultural systems. However, I do not think this is a reason to reject the scientific project altogether – partly because better and more rigorous science is how we can overcome such biases. And this leads to improved knowledge of our origins. As Knight writes when discussing the founders and pioneers of modern anthropology:

> Enlightenment was an end in itself; their own new science was an important aspect of the gradually advancing self-awareness of humankind. The idea of

debating whether this self-awareness was 'useful' would not have occurred to them. And indeed, it was only after the science of culture had isolated itself from almost all related branches of science and had *ceased to ask itself fundamental questions* that such an idea could have arisen.

(Knight 1995: 63)

The notion of developmental stages from our prehistoric hunter-gatherer ancestors through the growth of civilisations to the modern technological nation state, is central to Jung's psychological theory of human history. Without this developmental model, the entire edifice of analytical psychological and its unique contribution to socio-logical and historical analysis, crumbles. For example, Jung argued that many of the psychological conditions suffered by modern humans, result from the breakdown of intimate family units of the kind that would have characterised most of our evolution-ary history. These small endogamous units and the associated emotional intimacy were, in Jung's view, increasingly abandoned as exogamous systems expanded with the growth of civilisations and the associated increase in population.

Such an approach can be found throughout Jung's writings. However, the most extensive treatment of the issue is in *The Psychology of Transference* (Jung 1983: 63–72). In this work, Jung uses Spencer and Gillen as well as the English Jungian anthropologist John Layard (1891–1974) as sources. Jung's analysis is a classic example of anthropological stage theory and Morgan's Enlightenment mandate 'to explore the Universal History of Mankind' (Fox 2011: 318). Jung assumes that prehistoric social organisation was characterised by endogamy and that it was fo-cussed on the emotional ties of the immediate family or kin group; as he writes: '[i] ncest, as an endogamous relationship, is an expression of the libido which serves to hold the family together' (Jung 1983: 62). However, with expanding social net-works and the eventual the growth of civilisations and the accompanying increase in population, the endogamous tendency was increasingly replaced by exogamous marriage systems.

In developing these ideas, Jung quotes Spencer and Gillen, who wrote that ex-ogamy serves to 'bind more or less closely together groups of individuals who are mutually interested in one another's welfare' a system which has 'been one of the most powerful agents in the early stages of the upward development of the human race' (Spencer and Gillen 1904: 74). As Jung elaborates:

In the interests of the welfare and development of the tribe, the exogamous so-cial order thrust the endogamous tendency into the background so as to prevent the danger of regression to a state of having no groups at all. It insisted on the introduction of "new blood" both physically and spiritually, and it thus proved to be a powerful instrument in the development of culture.

(Jung 1983: 66)

Exogamy, or mating outside the immediate group, is a central feature of the social structure hunter-gatherer communities, with primates even showing an incipient form of this tendency. However, in hunter-gatherer cultures exogamy is often in a state of tension with endogamous principles and the desire to reside with immediate family. For example, a woman may feel a sense of tension between her attachment to her own siblings and parents and her husband and his kin group. There may be an emotional tendency to seek attachment to, and the associated protection, of family and close kin – however the need for the group to establish alliances with other groups may mean she resides with her husband more than she would like. Endogamous or incestuous tendencies seem to be associated with blood symbolism as well as serpent imagery, motifs that both Jungians and Knight and colleagues highlight. I explore these associations in greater detail in the chapters that follow.

One of the important features of this configuration is that a woman will have relations in two groups – for example, in one group her brother and matrilineal kin and in the other group her husband and his kin. Such forms of 'supragroup levels of social organization' result in reduced conflict between groups – for example, the men in the women's kin group are less likely to attack the group where she resides with her husband, as attacking that group would potentially endanger a member of their own family (Chapais 2010). Another benefit is that the federations formed by exogamous marriage exchange means that the two groups will have reciprocal hunting rights in each other's territory. This is particularly important for hunter-gatherer communities living in desert ecologies that are subject to capricious fluctuations in rainfall. Jung comments on this phenomenon when he avers that cross-cousin marriage

> … represented an archetype that combined exogamy and endogamy in the most fortunate way, for while it prevented marriage between brother and sister it provided a substitute in the cross-cousin marriage. This relationship is still close enough to satisfy the endogamous tendency more or less, but distant enough to include other groups and to extend the orderly cohesion of the tribe.
>
> (Jung 1983: 70)

Commenting on this phenomenon in his book *Primeval Kinship: How Pair-bonding Gave Birth to Human Society*, Bernard Chapais writes:

> From an evolutionary perspective, the nature of bonds between siblings in our species appears to be the single most original characteristic of human kinship. A particularly puzzling phenomenon is the importance of the brother–sister bond in so many human societies. The brother–sister kinship complex integrates phenomena like the avunculate—the special relationship between a brother, his sister, and the sister's son—cross-cousin marriage prescriptions, and various kinship terminologies. The brother–sister kinship complex has no equivalent in nonhuman primates. Not only is it uniquely human, it is a cornerstone of human society's deep structure.
>
> (Chapais 2009: 202)

It is the dynamic between emotional attachment to kin and exogamous marriage that, according to Robin Fox, underpins myths about incest, as well as its actual occurrence among, for example, the royal families of ancient Egypt. As he avers:

> This tension is expressed, then, in the two extremes of the sibling incest story. The first one is where an ideal union is formed (or at least desired) that excludes outsiders and dodges the demands of exogamy, and the other where the relationship is one of unwanted sex, usually forced by the brother but sometimes initiated by the sister. In between is the situation where the two bonds are in a state of conflict and the sisters are pulled both ways: toward brothers and kin, and toward husband and in-laws.
>
> (Fox 2011: 141)

Jung argued that the endogamous tendency was associated with the unconscious, his rationale assumingly being that such an attraction to the small and immediate family group was based more on primary affects than the conscious personality (Jung 1983: 67). Be that as it may, from this assumption he inferred that incest stories of the kind Fox alluded to could become actualised in real life but only by royalty. As he writes when discussing the royal incest prerogative of the ancient Egyptians, we see instances of 'human figures who have the power to do what others may not do—kings and princes, for example' (Jung 1983: 67). This anthropologically informed analysis of kinship, endogamy and exogamy, is the basis of Jung's conception of the alchemical divine marriage in *The Psychology of Transference* (Jung 1983: 63–72). What the above discussion demonstrates is that without the notion of historical development and anthropologically informed stage theory, Jung's conception of alchemy is deprived of its sociological basis.

For Jung, the growth of population that occurred with the development of civilisation 'led to a further extension of the exogamous order' (Jung 1983: 69). He argues that as a consequence, the endogamous tendency of kinship libido was forced into the background of social life, with the repression of the sentiments associated with our more intimate archaic social structure being implicated in the 'psychic dissociation of collective man' (Jung 1983: 71). As he elaborates:

> While exogamy was limited by endogamy, it resulted in a natural organization of society which has entirely disappeared today. Everyone is now a stranger among strangers. Kinship libido—which could still engender a satisfying feeling of belonging together, as for instance in the early Christian communities—has long been deprived of its object. But, being an instinct, it is not to be satisfied by any mere substitute such as a creed, party, nation, or state. It wants the *human* connection. That is the core of the whole transference phenomenon, and it is impossible to argue it away, because relationship to the self is at once relationship to our fellow man, and no one can be related to the latter until he is related to himself.
>
> (Jung 1983: 71–2)

Jung's conception of human historical development, from small-scale hunter-gatherers, through the growth of civilisations, to the mass aggregation of human beings in the modern nation state, forms the basis of his analysis of modern human culture. The repression of the endogamous tendency of the immediate, small-scale family group creates a sense of inner disquiet that can be harnessed by demagogues who 'attempt to unite a socially and psychologically fractured polity through appeal to our more ancient yet repressed social instincts' (Clark 2020: 148). As Jung writes, the ensuing sense of absence is often filled by 'tin gods with totalitarian pretensions who call themselves State or Fuehrer' – a process that gives rise to a 'totalitarian psychosis with its frightful consequences and the intolerable disturbance of human relationships' (Jung 1983: 69). Jung's diagnosis reminds us of Hannah Arendt's analysis of twentieth-century totalitarianism: '… loneliness has become an everyday experience of the ever-growing masses of our century. The merciless process into which totalitarianism drives and organises the masses looks like a suicidal escape from this reality' (Arendt 1973: 478).

There is some very suggestive evidence supportive of Jung's contention that the historical breakdown of the immediate, endogamous kin group may be implicated in various forms of psychosocial dysfunction. It is important to note that one of the assertions of kinship theory is that ancestral grandmothers provided much of the extra metabolic and social support necessary for the increase in brain and body size in the hominin lineage we see some 2 million years ago with the emergence of *Homo erectus* – the so-called grandmother hypothesis of human evolution (O'Connell, Hawkes, and Blurton Jones 1999; Hrdy 2009; Hawkes and Coxworth 2013). One of the implications of this theory is that if young mothers in modern societies are deprived of the social supports and access to kinship networks that characterised our deep evolutionary past, then they may be subject to high levels of psychosocial stress.

For example, children and mothers have been found to have lower stress hormone levels when they have extended support networks of the kind that would have been common in our evolutionary past (Flinn and Leone 2006; Balaji et al. 2007; Kramer 2010; Gettler et al. 2021). These findings are particularly relevant to mothers in modern industrial societies who may lack the support network of immediate kin of the kind our ancestors would have enjoyed. Such lack of support seems to produce numerous psychosocial stresses, which also impacts infant and child development. This is just one example of how a *depth sociology* inspired by Jung's anthropologically informed historical and cultural analysis may be germane to modern research endeavours.

Robert Storey has made similar observations to Jung in regard to the rapid historical transition from our ancient hunter-gatherer kin based systems to the modern state. For Storey, the demographic transformations of modernity are characterised by 'the depersonalization of our social exchanges and the weakening of our ties with family and friends, especially with parents and siblings.' By understanding the breakdown of such ancient kinship structures

… the familiarly Kafkaesque angst of our age begins to find its focus. Emotionally and psychologically, ours is the disquiet of the late-Pleistocene hominid thrust into a crowd of alien bipeds-on-the-make and dependent on the kindness of strangers.

(Storey 1996: 60)

The above discussion suggests ways in which Jung's conception of historical development may be refined in terms of current research into the evolution of kinship structures. In his analysis of our unique suite of social and familial structures, the entire combination of which exists in no other primate species, Chapais has developed what he calls a 'comparative sociology of human and nonhuman primates' (Chapais 2009: 11). A Jungian extension of the evolutionary ideas of Chapais, Fox, Knight and others would represent a comparative *depth sociology* of human and nonhuman primates.

Ontogeny and Phylogeny: Jung and the Evolution of Consciousness

One of the most important aspects of Jung's evolutionary anthropology was his view that there was a parallel between the development of consciousness during phylogeny or evolution of the species and that of ontogeny or development of the individual. However, this did not mean, as it is often mistakenly assumed, that Jung believed archaic hominins were the equivalent of children. What he did argue is that in individual development, and also throughout the process of hominin evolution, we see a transition from affect-based subcortical brain systems to ones based on consciousness and an individualised sense of self or ego (Clark 2021, 2022, 2023).

This hypothesis represented the psychological aspect of Jung's broader conception of humankind's evolutionary development – that is the psychological dimension of the developmental stages theory central to nineteenth and early twentieth-century anthropology. For Jung, the historical development from Pleistocene hunter-gatherers, through the agricultural or Neolithic revolution, the emergence of city states and the growth of civilisations, to the modern scientific world, was characterised by increasing differentiation of consciousness. This process of differentiation was accompanied in Jung's view by increasing levels of dissociation from unconscious processes – a split that analytical psychology seeks to heal (Jung 2014b: 253–64).

Nietzsche, in addition to the *Naturphilosophen*, was one of the influences on Jung's thinking regarding these issues. For example, in *Human, All to Human*, Nietzsche develops a theory about the relationship between dreaming and our evolutionary history. He argues that during earlier stages of evolution, conscious experience had more affinity with dream states and forms of hallucinatory experience than it did in later periods; as he writes: '... dream-ideas ... [remind] us again of earlier mankind in which hallucinations were extraordinarily frequent.' He goes on to add that 'in our sleep and dreams, we go through the work of earlier mankind once more' (Nietzsche 1994: 20). Nietzsche associates this form of archaic dreamlike thinking with the 'poet' and 'artist' who 'reminds us of an older mankind, and can help us understand it.' He contrasts this mode of thinking with the more recent development of 'acute logical thinking' (Nietzsche 1994: 22). As he elaborates:

I think that man still draws conclusions in his dreams as mankind once did *in a waking state* ... This old aspect of humanity lives on in our dreams, for it is the basis upon which higher reason developed and is still developing, in every human: the dream restores us to distant states of human culture and gives us a means to understand them better.

(Nietzsche 1994: 21)

Importantly for Nietzsche dreaming has a restorative function, one that is particularly important for those living in cultures characterised by acute logical thinking; as he writes, dreaming is a 'recuperation for a brain which must satisfy by day the stricter demands on thought made by higher culture' (Nietzsche 1994: 20).

In *Symbols of Transformation*, Jung quotes from these passages of Nietzsche adding the notion that the pre-logical or pre-theoretical thinking of infants and young children may have affinities with earlier stages of human evolutionary history:

This idea is not at all strange: we know it quite well from comparative anatomy and from evolution, which show that the structure and function of the human body are the result of a series of embryonic mutations corresponding to similar mutations in our racial history. The supposition that there may also be in psychology a correspondence between ontogenesis and phylogenesis therefore seems justified. If this is so it would mean that infantile thinking and dream thinking are simply a recapitulation of earlier evolutionary stages.

(Jung 2014d: 23)

We can see here that Jung synthesised Nietzsche's ideas with the evolutionary developmental theories of the *Naturphilosophen*. It is also important to note that Jung is not claiming that archaic humans were the equivalent of children. What he is arguing is that dream and infantile thinking may be both expressions of ancient brain systems – that is primary process affect-based systems that in both ontogeny and phylogeny develop before the emergence of ego consciousness (Clark 2022, 2023).

The notion that dream-like thinking may have characterised the waking state of our ancestors is not so strange as it may first seem. Interestingly, the idea does find some support from the neuroscientific study of dreaming. For example, it has been proposed that dreams are manifestations of ancient primary process affective brain systems (Hobson 1999; Hobson and Voss 2011; Hobson 2014; Carhart-Harris et al. 2014). In his pioneering *Affective Neuroscience: The Foundations of Human and Animal Emotions*, Jaak Panksepp makes a similar argument. For example, he suggests that people who hold dream experiences in great esteem 'may be correctly affirming the importance of the affective information that is encoded through our ancient emotional urges for the proper conduct of our waking activities' (Panksepp 2004: 135).

Elaborating on this idea, Panksepp suggests that prior to the emergence of complex cognitive strategies, 'animals may have generated most of their behaviour from primary-process psychobehavioral routines that we now recognize as the primitive emotional systems.' Over evolutionary time, these primitive systems, in Panksepp's view, were superseded by more sophisticated forms of cognition 'that required not only more neocortex but also new arousal mechanisms to sustain efficient waking functions within those emerging brain areas.' The evolution of these systems, such as those subserving thalamocortical cognitive mechanisms, may have resulted in 'the old emotional arousal system' assuming a subsidiary role such as 'doing computations on the environmental relationships that had transpired during waking, especially those with a strong emotional content.' Summarising this view, he argues the period of rapid eye movement sleep (REM) during which dreaming occurs may have controlled – as Nietzsche suggested – the waking lives of our ancestors:

> ... what is now known as the REM mechanism [may have] originally controlled a primitive form of waking arousal. With the evolution of higher brain areas, a newer and more efficient waking mechanism may have been needed, leading to the emergence of [the system of waking arousal]. The more ancient form of arousal may have been gradually overridden and relegated to providing a back-ground function such as the integration of emotional information that seems to occur during dreaming.
>
> (Panksepp 2004: 135)

As I outlined in Chapter 1, Haeckel had a significant impact on the development of evolutionary embryology in the nineteenth and twentieth centuries, influence which continues to this day (Hoßfeld and Olsson 2003). He also had a profound influence on developmental psychology in the twentieth century from Freud and Jung to Piaget (Bair 2003: 215, 718 and 20; Koops 2012, 2015; Cambray 2014, 2017), influence that is evident in Jung's interpretative gloss of Nietzsche.

In her *Organic Memory: History and the Body in the Late Nineteenth and Early Twentieth Centuries*, Laura Otis argues that Haeckel's 'biogenetic law' and the concept of recapitulation, underpinned racist conceptions that so-called primitive races were on a 'lower' rung of the evolutionary hierarchy. Consequently, Africans, for example, came to represent an intermediate form between Europeans and humanity's animal ancestors. Such a schemata 'implied that the present organism contained its past within it, and that one could thus read phylogeny, or ancestral development, by observing ontogeny, or individual development' (Otis 1994: 8). This framework, according to Otis, underpinned both Freud's and Jung's evolutionary model of the psyche and the 'Haeckelian ... parallel of the mental patient, the child, the primitive ancestor, and the contemporary "primitive" person' (Otis 1994: 208). Otis argues that the relationship between ontogeny and phylogeny developed by Haeckel and early developmental embryologists enjoyed 'immense popularity in the late nineteenth century' but that consequently it was 'rejected by biology in the mid-twentieth century' (Otis 1994: 5).

Numerous Jungian scholars have made similar arguments, suggesting that Jung's reliance on Haeckel's notion of the relationship between ontogeny and phylogeny, and his supposedly discredited 'biogenetic law' means that Jung's evolutionary conception of human psychology is invalid (Fordham 1957: 22 and 30; Shamdasani 2003: 266–7). Additionally, it has also been argued that Jung's use of Haeckel's' 'biogenetic law' resulted in him equating ancestral adults with modern children (Dalal 1988: 273–4).

These critiques are based on a number of misconceptions. Firstly, the above authors claim Haeckel's biogenetic law has been discredited by the scientific community. This is not the case – Haeckel's ideas are still considered relevant by evolutionary developmental biologists (Richardson and Keuck 2002; Hoßfeld and Olsson 2003; Laubichler and Maienschein 2007; Olsson, Levit, and Hoßfeld 2017). Secondly, the notion that ontogeny recapitulates phylogeny was only one rare example of a multitude of relationships between ontogeny and phylogeny analysed by Haeckel – many of which did not in fact involve recapitulation of ancestral adult stages in the ontogeny of extant species (Richardson and Keuck 2002; Olsson et al. 2017). For example, the 'biogenetic law' included new stages within embryological development, addition of stages at the end of development and various forms of heterochrony (Gould 1977; Richardson and Keuck 2002: 209–11). Haeckel's concept of heterochrony (Greek for different times) sought to explain how the growth of different parts of an organism could be altered in relation to one another, giving rise to different species, a concept that is central to modern theories of human evolution (Minugh-Purvis and McNamara 2002; Clark and Henneberg 2015).

Jung was perfectly aware of these distinctions, explicitly arguing against the notion that a modern child passes through the evolutionary stages of our ancestors, and that consequently our ancestors were the equivalent of a child. As he writes of the archaic ancestors of modern humans, just as those 'first fishy ancestors of man, with their gill slits, were not embryos, but fully developed creatures, so the myth making and myth inhabiting man was a grown reality and not a four year old child' (Jung 2014d: 24–5). What Jung is arguing is that different species may evolve from a common ancestor through alteration of embryological and developmental processes, but that does not mean the juveniles of such descendent species are equivalent to the adults of the ancestral population from which they evolved. What are often similar are the earliest stages of embryogenesis with the differences developing as ontogenetic trajectories are alerted from this underlying shared genetic and somatic substrate (Clark 2023: 12–13).

Jung's nuanced understanding of the relationship between developmental processes and evolution is also one of the reasons he distanced himself from Freud's incest theory. While the criticism of the biogenetic law by the above authors is to some degree accurate, particularly in regard to Freud, Jung was actually at pains to distance himself from the notion and the connections Freud made with his theory of incest. For example, when discussing the 'concretism of Freudian theory' Jung questions the explanation of primitive ritual in terms of Freud's incest theory. While such rituals may represent a transition to more primitive primary process brain systems this does not mean those who participate in them are the psychological equivalent of a child. Jung made this distinction when discussing Australian Indigenous rituals and the affinities such rites have with similar practices in other cultures:

> This atavistic identification with human and animal ancestors can be interpreted psychologically as an integration of the unconscious, a veritable bath of renewal in the life-source where one is once again a fish, unconscious as in sleep, intoxication, and death. Hence the sleep of incubation, the Dionysian orgy, and the ritual death in initiation. Naturally the proceedings always take place in some hallowed spot.
>
> (Jung 1980: 131)

Jung goes on to argue that we could interpret such rites in terms of Freudian theory and that the *temenos* or scared space of ritual activity would then be 'the womb of the mother and the rite a regression to incest.' He goes on to reject this notion arguing that such rites 'cannot possibly be explained as a mere regression to infantilism. Otherwise the highest and most important achievements of mankind would ultimately be nothing but the perverted wishes of children, and the word "childish" would have lost its *raison d'etre*' (Jung 1980: 131). Jung continues, stating that the symbolism 'of the rites of renewal, if taken seriously, points far beyond the merely archaic and infantile to man's innate psychic disposition, which is the result and deposit of all ancestral life right down to the animal level' (Jung 1980: 134). It is clear from the above discussion that Jung did not equate early humans with the psychology of children.

While Freud saw incest as literal desire for sex, Jung saw it as the expression of a more general emotional orientation – what he called 'kinship libido' (Jung 1983: 62). Brodersen has discussed these issues, noting that Freud *literalises* incest as a regressive developmental phenomenon, whereas Jung interpreted it as a wider symbolic desire to unite with unconscious potential. In this sense, it is crucial to the individuation process facilitating 'affect regulation, free will and independent thinking' rather than being viewed as a tabooed sexual instinct. As she elaborates:

> Jung's interpretation of incest emphasises its *symbolic* nature. Jung uses incest as a metaphor for fusion with unconscious creative processes whereby fusion with the contrasexual other brings forward a rebirth of potential, rather than acts as a concrete sexualised outer relationship.
>
> (Brodersen 2019: 85)

From this perspective, incest is an expression of primary process affect that originally evolved in the small intimate family structure of the Pleistocene. As culture expanded and civilisations developed, those affects were redirected to facilitate other bonds in the expanding exogamous social structures of more recent times. They also served as the basis of cultural symbolism and various forms of ritual practice. Jung does not conceive of such regression to ancient primary process brain systems as a form of infantilism, but as adults integrating phylogenetically ancient brain systems with the more recently evolved conscious ego. Jung's connection between dreamlife, mythological or symbolic thinking, and early evolutionary stages evident in his gloss on Nietzsche's comment, seeks to highlight activation of ancient brain systems in both dreamlife and mythological thinking – not that early humans were the mental equivalent of a child.

In his theory of the emergence of consciousness, Jung integrated various strands of knowledge, from fossil science and anthropology to the relationship between ontogeny and phylogeny. He developed a theory to explain modern forms of individual and collective psychopathology, which he suggested resulted from the suppression of ancient endogamous tendencies in modern human populations. This evolutionary model focussed on historical development from our small-scale hunter-gatherer ancestors, through the growth of civilisations to the modern secular state. This developmental stage theory, growing out of nineteenth-century anthropology and fused with the theory of ontogeny and phylogeny developed by the *Naturphilosophen*, is the theoretical foundation upon which analytical psychology is built.

References

Arendt, H. 1973. *The Origins of Totalitarianism* (Harcourt Brace Jovanovich).
Bachofen, J.J. 1967. *Myth, Religion, and Mother Right: Selected Writings of J. J. Bachofen* (Routledge).
Bair, D. 2003. *Jung: A Biography* (Little Brown).
Balaji, A.B., A.H. Claussen, D.C. Smith, S.N. Visser, M.J. Morales, and R. Perou. 2007. 'Social Support Networks and Maternal Mental Health and Well-Being', *Journal of Women's Health (Larchmt)*, 16: 1386–96.
Bhandar, B. 2018. *Colonial Lives of Property: Law, Land, and Racial Regimes of Ownership* (Duke University Press).
Bowler, J., H. Johnston, J.M. Olley, J.R. Prescott, R.G. Roberts, W. Shawcross, et al. 2003. 'New Ages for Human Occupation and Climatic Change at Lake Mungo, Australia', *Nature*, 421: 837–40.
Briffault, R. 1927. *The Mothers: A Study of the Origins of Sentiments and Institutions* (Macmillan).
Brodersen, E. 2019. *Taboo, Personal and Collective Representations: Origin and Positioning within Cultural Complexes* (Taylor & Francis).
Burston, D. 1991. *The Legacy of Erich Fromm* (Harvard University Press).
Cambray, J. 2014. 'Romanticism and Revolution in Jung's Science.' in Jones, R.A. (ed.), *Jung and the Question of Science* (Routledge).
Cambray, J. 2017. 'The Red Book: Entrances and Exits.' in Kirsch, T., and G. Hogenson (eds.), *The Red Book: Reflections on CG Jung's Liber Novus* (Routledge).
Carhart-Harris, R.L., and K.J. Friston. 2010. 'The Default-Mode, Ego-Functions and Free-Energy: A Neurobiological Account of Freudian Ideas', *Brain*, 133: 1265–83.
Carhart-Harris, R.L., R. Leech, P.J. Hellyer, M. Shanahan, A. Feilding, E. Tagliazucchi, et al. 2014. 'The Entropic Brain: A Theory of Conscious States Informed by Neuroimaging Research with Psychedelic Drugs', *Frontiers in Human Neuroscience*, 8: 1–22.
Carter, P. 2013. *The Road to Botany Bay: An Exploration of Landscape and History* (University of Minnesota Press).

Chapais, B. 2009. *Primeval Kinship: How Pair-Bonding Gave Birth to Human Society* (Harvard University Press).

Chapais, B. 2010. 'The Deep Structure of Human Society: Primate Origins and Evolution.' in Kappeler, P.M., and J. Silk (eds.), *Mind the Gap: Tracing the Origins of Human Universals* (Springer Berlin Heidelberg).

Clark, G. 2020. 'Carl Jung, John Layard and Jordan Peterson: Assessing Theories of Human Social Evolution and Their Implications for Analytical Psychology', *International Journal of Jungian Studies*, 12: 129–58.

Clark, G. 2021. 'Carl Jung and the Psychedelic Brain: An Evolutionary Model of Analytical Psychology Informed by Psychedelic Neuroscience', *International Journal of Jungian Studies*, 14(2): 1–30.

Clark, G. 2022. 'The Dionysian Primate: Goethe, Nietzsche, Jung and Psychedelic Neuroscience.' in Miils, J., and D. Burston (eds.), *Psychoanalysis and the Mind-Body Problem* (Routledge).

Clark, G. 2023. 'Rethinking Jung's Reception of Kant and the Naturphilosophen: Archetypes, Evolutionary Developmental Biology and the Future of Analytical Psychology', *International Journal of Jungian Studies*, 1: 1–31.

Clark, G., and M. Henneberg. 2015. 'The Life History of Ardipithecus ramidus: A Heterochronic Model of Sexual and Social Maturation', *Anthropological Review*, 78: 109–32.

Dalal, Farhad. 1988. 'Jung: A Racist', *British Journal of Psychotherapy*, 4: 263–79.

Derrida, J. 2016. *Of Grammatology* (Johns Hopkins University Press).

Diogo, R. 2024. *Darwin's Racism, Sexism, and Idolization: Their Tragic Societal and Scientific Repercussions* (Springer Nature Switzerland).

Durkheim, É. 2008. *The Elementary Forms of Religious Life* (OUP Oxford).

Elkin, A.P. 1993. *Aboriginal Men of High Degree: Initiation and Sorcery in the World's Oldest Tradition* (Inner Traditions/Bear).

Ellenberger, H.F. 1970. *The Discovery of the Unconscious: The History and Evolution of Dynamic Psychiatry* (Basic Books).

Engels, F. 2010. *The Origin of the Family, Private Property and the State* (Penguin Books Limited).

Flinn, M., and D. Leone. 2006. 'Early Family Trauma and the Ontogeny of Glucocorticoid Stress Response in the Human Child: Grandmother as a Secure Base', *Journal of Developmental Processes*, 1: 31–68.

Fordham, M. 1957. *New Developments in Analytical Psychology* (Routledge and K. Paul).

Foucault, M. 2005. *The Order of Things* (Taylor & Francis).

Foucault, M. 2013. *History of Madness* (Taylor & Francis).

Fox, R. 1980. *The Red Lamp of Incest* (Dutton).

Fox, R. 2011. *The Tribal Imagination: Civilization and the Savage Mind* (Harvard University Press).

Freud, S. 2012. *Totem and Taboo* (Taylor & Francis).

Freud, S., C.G. Jung, and W. McGuire. 1974. *The Freud/Jung Letters: The Correspondence between Sigmund Freud and C. G. Jung. Edited by William McGuire* (Princeton University Press).

Gardner, L., and F. Gray. 2016. *Feminist Views from Somewhere: Post-Jungian Themes in Feminist Theory* (Taylor & Francis).

Gettler, L., S. Lew-Levy, M. Sarma, V. Miegakanda, M. Doxsey, J. Meyer, et al. 2021. 'Children's Fingernail Cortisol among BaYaka Foragers of the Congo Basin: Associations with Fathers' Roles', *Philosophical Transactions of the Royal Society B*, 376: 20200031.

Gillen, F.J., D.J. Mulvaney, H. Morphy, and A. Petch. 1997. *"My Dear Spencer": The Letters of F.J. Gillen to Baldwin Spencer* (Hyland House).

Goodwyn, E.D. 2014. 'Depth Psychology and Symbolic Anthropology: Toward a Depth Sociology of Psychocultural Interaction', *The International Journal for the Psychology of Religion*, 24: 169–84.

Gould, S.J. 1977. *Ontogeny and Phylogeny* (Belknap Press of Harvard University Press).

Gould, S.J. 1996. *The Mismeasure of Man* (Norton).

Greenwood, S. 2013. 'Emile Durkheim and C. G. Jung: Structuring a Transpersonal Sociology of Religion', *International Journal of Transpersonal Studies*, 32: 42–52.

Harding, M.E. 1936. *Woman's Mysteries: Ancient and Modern* (Longman).

Harris, M. 1968. *The Rise of Anthropological Theory: A History of Theories of Culture* (Routledge & Kegan Paul).

Hauke, C. 2000. *Jung and the Postmodern: The Interpretation of Realities* (Routledge).

Hawkes, K., and J.E. Coxworth. 2013. 'Grandmothers and the Evolution of Human Longevity: A Review of Findings and Future Directions', *Evolutionary Anthropology*, 22: 294–302.

Hobson, A. 1999. *Dreaming as Delirium: How the Brain Goes Out of Its Mind* (MIT Press).

Hobson, A. 2002. *The Dream Drugstore: Chemically Altered States of Consciousness* (MIT Press).

Hobson, A. 2014. *Psychodynamic Neurology: Dreams, Consciousness, and Virtual Reality* (Taylor & Francis).

Hobson, J.A., C.C.H. Hong, and K.J. Friston. 2014. 'Virtual Reality and Consciousness Inference in Dreaming', *Frontiers in Psychology*, 5: 1–18.

Hobson, A., and U. Voss. 2011. 'A Mind to Go Out of: Reflections on Primary and Secondary Consciousness', *Consciousness and Cognition*, 20: 993–7.

Hobson, J.A. 2009. 'REM Sleep and Dreaming: Towards a Theory of Protoconsciousness', *Nature Reviews Neuroscience*, 10: 803–13.

Hoßfeld, U., and L. Olsson. 2003. 'The Road from Haeckel: The Jena Tradition in Evolutionary Morphology and the Origins of "Evo-Devo"', *Biology and Philosophy*, 18: 285–307.

Hrdy, S.B. 2009. *Mothers and Others: The Evolutionary Origins of Mutual Understanding* (Belknap Press of Harvard University Press).

Hume, L. 2002. *Ancestral Power: The Dreaming, Consciousness and Aboriginal Australians* (Melbourne University Press).

Johnson, A.W., and T. Earle. 2022. *The Evolution of Human Societies: From Foraging Group to Agrarian State, Second Edition* (Stanford University Press).

Jung, C.G. 1953. *Collected Works of C. G. Jung, Volume 13: Alchemical Studies* (Princeton University Press).

Jung, C.G. 1970. *Mysterium Coniunctionis: An Inquiry into the Separation and Synthesis of Psychic Opposites in Alchemy* (Princeton University Press).

Jung, C.G. 1980. *Collected Works of C.G. Jung, Volume 12: Psychology and Alchemy* (Princeton University Press).

Jung, C.G. 1983. *The Psychology of the Transference* (Routledge).

Jung, C.G. 1989. *Memories, Dreams, Reflections* (Knopf Doubleday Publishing Group).

Jung, C.G. 1991. *Psychological Types* (Routledge).

Jung, C.G. 1998. *Visions: Notes of the Seminar Given in 1930-1934* (Routledge).

Jung, C.G. 2014a. *Collected Works of C.G. Jung, Volume 9 (Part 1): Archetypes and the Collective Unconscious* (Princeton University Press).

Jung, C.G. 2014b. *Collected Works of C.G. Jung, Volume 18: The Symbolic Life: Miscellaneous Writings* (Princeton University Press).

Jung, C.G. 2014c. *The Structure and Dynamics of the Psyche* (Taylor & Francis).

Jung, C.G. 2014d. *Symbols of Transformation* (Taylor & Francis).

Jung, C.G., and E. Neumann. 2015. *Analytical Psychology in Exile: The Correspondence of C. G. Jung and Erich Neumann* (Princeton University Press).

Knight, C. 1995. *Blood Relations: Menstruation and the Origins of Culture* (Yale University Press).

Knight, C. 2009. 'Early Human Kinship Was Matrilineal.' Nicholas J. Allen, Hilary Callan, Robin Dunbar, Wendy James in *Early Human Kinship* (Blackwell Publishing Ltd.).

Knight, C., and J. Lewis. 2016. 'Towards a Theory of Everything.' in Power, C., M. Finnegan, and H. Calla (eds.), *Human Origins: Contributions from Social Anthropology* (Berghahn Books).

Knight, C., and C. Power. 2005. 'Grandmothers, Politics, and Getting Back to Science.' in Chasiotis, A., W. Schiefenhöve, and E. Voland (eds.), *Grandmotherhood. The Evolutionary Significance of the Second Half of Female Life* (Rutgers University Press).

Knight, C. 1988. 'Menstrual Synchrony and the Australian Rainbow Snake.' in Buckley, T., and A. Gottlieb (eds.), *Blood Magic: The Anthropology of Menstruation* (University of California Press).

Koops, W. 2012. 'Jean Jacques Rousseau, Modern Developmental Psychology, and Education', *European Journal of Developmental Psychology*, 9: 46–56.

Koops, W. 2015. 'No Developmental Psychology without Recapitulation Theory', *European Journal of Developmental Psychology*, 12: 630–9.

Kramer, K. 2010. 'Cooperative Breeding and Its Significance to the Demographic Success of Humans', *Annual Review of Anthropology*, 39: 417–36.

Laubichler, M.D., and J. Maienschein. 2007. *From Embryology to Evo-Devo: A History of Developmental Evolution* (MIT Press).

Laughlin, C.D. 2011. *Communing with the Gods: Consciousness, Culture and the Dreaming Brain* (Daily Grail Publishing).

Lawson, T.T. 2008. *Carl Jung, Darwin of the Mind* (Karnac).

Lévy-Bruhl, L. 1983. *Primitive Mythology: The Mythic World of the Australian and Papuan Natives* (University of Queensland Press).

Lincoln, J.S. 1970. *The Dream in Primitive Cultures* (Johnson Reprint Corporation).

Lowie, R.H. 1987. *The History of Ethnological Theory* (George G. Harrap & Company).

Mayr, E. 1963. 'The Taxonomic Evaluation of Fossil Hominids.' in Washburn, S.L. (ed.), *Classification and Human Evolution* (Routledge).

McGregor, R. 2015. *Imagined Destinies: Aboriginal Australians and the Doomed Race Theory, 1880–1939* (Melbourne University Publishing).

Minugh-Purvis, N., and K.J. McNamara. 2002. *Human Evolution through Developmental Change* (Johns Hopkins University Press).

Morgan, L.H. 1985. *Ancient Society* (University of Arizona Press).

Morphy, H. 1997. "Gillen: Man of Science.' in Morphy, J., H. Mulvaney and A. Petch (eds.), *'My Dear Spencer': The Letters of F. J. Gillen to Baldwin Spencer* (Hyland House).

Morphy, H. 1988. 'Spencer and Gillen in Durkheim: The Theoretical Constructions of Ethnography.' in Allen, N.J., W.S.F. Pickering and W.W Miller (eds.), *On Durkheim's Elementary Forms of Religious Life* (Routledge).

Munn, N.D. 1973. *Walbiri Iconography: Graphic Representation and Cultural Symbolism in a Central Australian Society* (Cornell University Press).

Myers, F.R. 1991. *Pintupi Country, Pintupi Self: Sentiment, Place, and Politics among Western Desert Aborigines* (University of California Press).

Neumann, E. 1994. *The Fear of the Feminine: And Other Essays on Feminine Psychology* (Princeton University Press).

Neumann, E. 2015. *The Great Mother: An Analysis of the Archetype* (Princeton University Press).

Nietzsche, F. 1994. *Human, All Too Human* (Penguin Books Limited).

O'Connell, J.F., K. Hawkes, and N.G. Blurton Jones. 1999. 'Grandmothering and the Evolution of Homo erectus', *Journal of Human Evolution*, 36: 461–85.

Olsson, L., G.S. Levit, and U. Hoßfeld. 2017. 'The "Biogenetic Law" in Zoology: From Ernst Haeckel's Formulation to Current Approaches', *Theory in Biosciences*, 136: 19–29.

Otis, L. 1994. *Organic Memory: History and the Body in the Late Nineteenth & Early Twentieth Centuries* (University of Nebraska Press).

Pääbo, S. 2014. *Neanderthal Man: In Search of Lost Genomes* (Basic Books).

Panksepp, Jak 2004. *Affective Neuroscience: The Foundations of Human and Animal Emotions* (Oxford University Press).

Petchkovsky, L., C. Roque, and M. Beskow. 2003. 'Jung and the Dreaming: Analytical Psychology's Encounters with Aboriginal Culture', *Transcultural Psychiatry*, 40: 208–38.

Power, C. 2022. 'Lunarchy: The Original Human Economics of Time.' in Silva, F., and L. Henty (ed.), *Solarizing the Moon: Essays in Honour of Lionel Sims* (Archaeopress).

Power, C., M. Finnegan, and H. Callan. 2017. *Human Origins: Contributions from Social Anthropology* (Berghahn Books).

Power, C., V. Sommer, and I. Watts. 2013. 'The Seasonality Thermostat: Female Reproductive Synchrony and Male Behavior in Monkeys, Neanderthals, and Modern Humans', *PaleoAnthropology*, 2013: 33–60.

Power, C. 2017. 'Reconstructing a Source Cosmology for African Hunter-Gatherers.' in Power, C., M. Finnegan, and H. Calla (eds.), *Human Origins: Contributions from Social Anthropology* (Berghahn Books).

Richardson, M.K., and G. Keuck. 2002. 'Haeckel's ABC of Evolution and Development', *Biological Reviews of the Cambridge Philosophical Society*, 77: 495–528.

Rowland, S. 2004. 'Jung's Ghost Stories: Jung for Literary Theory in Feminism, Poststructuralism, and Postmodernism.' in Baumlin, J., T. Baumlin and G. Jensen (eds.), *Post-Jungian Criticism: Theory and Practice* (State University of New York Press).

Rowland, S. 2002. *Jung: A Feminist Revision* (Wiley).

Ryan, S. 1996. *The Cartographic Eye: How Explorers Saw Australia* (Cambridge University Press).

Said, E.W. 1995. *Orientalism* (Penguin Group).

Samuels, A. 2019. 'Notes on the Open Letter on Jung and "Africans" Published in the British Journal of Psychotherapy, November 2018', *Psychoanalysis, Culture & Society*, 24: 217–29.

Segal, R. 2007. 'Jung and Lévy-Bruhl', *Journal of Analytical Psychology*, 52: 635–58.

Shamdasani, S. 2003. *Jung and the Making of Modern Psychology: The Dream of a Science* (Cambridge University Press).

Spencer, B., and F.J. Gillen. 1904. *The Northern Tribes of Central Australia* (Macmillan and Company Limited).

Spencer, B., and F.J. Gillen. 2000. *The Native Tribes of Central Australia* (Adegi Graphics LLC).

Spencer, B., R.R. Marett, and T.K. Penniman. 1932. in Marett, R.R., K. Penniman (eds.), *Spencer's Scientific Correspondence* (Oxford University Press).

Stanner, W.E.H., and R. Manne 2011. *The Dreaming & Other Essays* (Schwartz Books Pty. Limited).

Staude, J.R. 1976. 'From Depth Psychology to Depth Sociology: Freud, Jung, and Lévi-Strauss', *Theory and Society*, 3: 303–38.

Stephens, L., D. Fuller, N. Boivin, T. Rick, N. Gauthier, and A. Kay, et al. 2019. 'Archaeological Assessment Reveals Earth's Early Transformation through Land Use', *Science*, 365: 897–902.

Storey, R. 1996. *Mimesis and the Human Animal: On the Biogenetic Foundations of Literary Representation* (Northwestern University Press).

Tacey, D. 2009. 'Mind and Earth: Psychic Influence beneath the Surface', *Jung Journal: Culture & Psyche*, 3: 15–32.

Watts, I. 2017. 'Rain Serpents in Northern Australia and Southern Africa: A Common Ancestry?' in Power, C., M. Finnegan and H. Callan (eds.), *Human Origins* (Berghahn Books).

Watts, I., M. Chazan, and J. Wilkins. 2016. 'Early Evidence for Brilliant Ritualized Display: Specularite Use in the Northern Cape (South Africa) between ~500 and ~300 Ka', *Current Anthropology*, 57: 287–310.

Way, A. 2022. 'Displacing History, Shifting Paradigms: Erasing Aboriginal Antiquity from Australian Anthropology', *History Australia*, 19: 710–30.

Chapter 3

Analytical Psychology and the Evolution of Sexual Dimorphism

Introduction

Sex-based differences between males and females and their putative biological basis have become contentious issues in contemporary Jungian scholarship. While Jung grounded his theory of anima and animus, and the associated concepts of Eros and Logos, in evolutionary biology, numerous Jungians have explicitly rejected this aspect of his thought. Jung argued that psychological differences between males and females are archetypal and have a deep evolutionary origin that precedes the emergence of consciousness. In this sense, they are foundational aspects of human psychological life. While this aspect of Jung's thought has been subject to extensive critique from feminist, postmodern and poststructuralist perspectives, there is also a strong element in Jungian scholarship that accepts his notion of biologically sex-based differences.

In this chapter, I discuss these different orientations and their relative merits. While there is a case to be made that some of Jung's views of men and women were influenced by his cultural background and its sexist assumptions, his general theory of sex-based psychological differences remains valid. More specifically, contemporary research in anthropology, psychology, comparative primatology and neuroscience all point to the conclusion that there are average differences in crucial aspects of male and female psychology and behaviour. However, given these differences are averages, there is also great deal of overlap between the sexes with many females exhibiting male-typical traits and many males female-typical traits.

The most pronounced aspect of human sexual dimorphism is in physical strength, which is related to pubertal development of muscle mass and bone density in males. This may be the physical correlate of psychological differences between males and females, with ancestral males having greater upper body strength for hunting and group protection from external threat. Such a hypothesis also explains sex-based differences in psychology.

DOI: 10.4324/9781032624549-4

Genes, Sex and the Evolution of Libido

When discussing the relationship between his anima theory and sex-based genes, Jung writes:

> Just as every individual derives from masculine and feminine genes, and the sex is determined by the predominance of the corresponding genes, so in the psyche it is only the conscious mind, in a man, that has the masculine sign, while the unconscious is by nature feminine. The reverse is true in the case of a woman. All I have done in my anima theory is to rediscover and reformulate this fact. It had long been known.
>
> (Jung 2014a: 175)

Elsewhere, when commenting on the genetic basis of human psychology, Jung writes that 'libido is appetite in its natural state' arguing that from 'the genetic point of view it is bodily needs like hunger, thirst, sleep, and sex, and emotional states or affects, which constitute the essence of libido' (Jung 2014c: 135–6). However, for Jung, the function of libido changes over the course of evolution, becoming utilised in very different ways. As he writes:

> As we know, an important change occurred in the principles of propagation during the ascent through the animal kingdom: the vast numbers of gametes which chance fertilization made necessary were progressively reduced in favour of assured fertilization and effective protection of the young. The decreased production of ova and spermatozoa set free considerable quantities of energy which soon sought and found new outlets.
>
> (Jung 2014c: 136)

What Jung is referring to here is one of the most important concepts in evolutionary theory – what is essentially the difference between quantity and quality in sexually reproducing species. Evolutionary biologists make a distinction between asexual and sexual reproduction. Asexual reproduction involves the creation of an exact replica of an organism with the same genetic material. Bacteria are an example of such a method of reproduction. Sexual reproduction, however, involves the combination of the genetic material of two individuals – one with sperm cells and the other with ova. The emergence of sexual reproduction, which is believed to be over 1 billion years old, has numerous benefits over asexual reproduction. One of the most important is that the combined genetic material of two individuals results in progeny possessing unique genetic material. This process, what biologists call genetic recombination, is one of the most important factors in the evolution of life on earth. The creation of unique genetic variants through recombination, along with other factors such as mutations, gives rise to the variation necessary for natural selection to occur. It is such variation, when sifted over millions of years by natural selection, that results in new species evolving. If it were not for such a process, early mammals would not have evolved from their reptilian ancestors some 200 million years ago; nor would have primates evolved from mammals. In fact, without the very ancient process of sexual reproduction, I would not be writing, nor would you be reading, this book about evolution and analytical psychology.

This very ancient form of reproduction means that there are two specific kinds of individuals in sexually reproducing species – that is, male and female (Geary 2010). Such species are ubiquitous, ranging from flowers to elephants and humans. This gives rise to the phenomenon of sexual dimorphism which can be found in many different forms and degrees throughout nature. For example, sexual dimorphism is not only evident in differences in reproductive biology; it also manifests itself in differences in body size, shape and strength, as well as behaviour and psychology. The evolutionary origin of sexual dimorphism in humans, and how it compares with other primates and mammals, is one of the central concerns of contemporary evolutionary theory.

What Jung is referring to when he mentions vast numbers of gametes and chance fertilisation is the form of sexual reproduction we see in many plant and marine species. In plants the male gamete or sperm is released in the form of pollen, which then combines with the female gamete or ovule in another plant. This results in the formation of an embryo which develops into a seed and consequently a new plant with unique genetic variation arising from sexual recombination. In many fish species a similar process of chance fertilisation occurs where large numbers of sperm and ova are released into the water with only a small number resulting in fertilisation and the survival of offspring into adulthood and sexual maturity. The important point in such cases is that large numbers of gametes and offspring are produced, but very little parental care is involved during the process of maturation. Additionally, only a small number will survive and go on to reach adulthood themselves. It is a reproductive strategy that prioritises quantity of gamete and offspring production over quality of parental care.

One of the major transitions in the evolutionary history of life on earth was from ancient reptiles to mammals some 200 million years ago. Mammals are characterised by the presence of milk-producing mammary glands. Such glands enable the mother to feed her young and increase the amount of care and nutrition offered each individual offspring. When contrasting mammals with the reproductive strategy evident in plants and fish, we can see that mammals essentially invert the process of chance fertilisation mentioned by Jung; that is, as opposed to a large number of offspring being produced, with minimal parental care, mammals produce fewer offspring but focus much more on nurturing, feeding and protecting those offspring. A similar strategy was adopted by birds. However, as opposed to nursing and feeding their young with milk-producing glands, birds will build a nest and provide food for their nestlings.

In many mammal and bird species, the increase in maternal care is associated with a phenomenon referred to as altriciality. The word altrical derives from the Latin *alere* which means to nurse, to rear or to nourish. Altricial offspring are essentially born immature and consequently they require an extended period of care and protection from the mother – although as we will see other individuals in addition to the mother (allomothers or alloparents) may also be involved in the care of young in some species, our own being a prime example. We can see examples of altriciality in our domestic dogs and cats; for example, they are born without hair, their eyes may still not have opened and they may be immobile and completely dependent on parental care for food, warmth and protection. Other mammals tend to be more pre-cocial and are able to move independently not long after birth; think, for example, of horses with their foals being able to walk independently soon after birth.

Humans are an altricial species; that is, human infants are born in a state extreme immaturity and helplessness and require intensive and prolonged maternal care. It is this evolutionary trend that Jung is referring to in the above passage where he stated that '… vast numbers of gametes which chance fertilization made necessary were progressively reduced in favour of assured fertilization and effective protection of the young' (Jung 2014c: 136).

It is important to emphasise that the transition from chance fertilisation and the production of a large number of offspring, to an increasing amount parental care, forms the basis of Jung's evolutionary conception of libido. Above, I mentioned Jung's notion that libido consists of emotional states or affects associated with bodily needs such as hunger, sleep and sex. He also links his conception of libido to nest building and increased care of the young. As he writes, 'libido which was originally employed in the production of ova and spermatozoa' became 'firmly organized in the function of nest-building' (Jung 2014c: 136). Such evolutionary transitions, according to Jung, resulted in libidinal energy being redirected to not only increased care of the young, but eventually artistic creation. As he avers:

> Thus we find the first stirrings of the artistic impulse in animals, but subservi-ent to the reproductive instinct and limited to the breeding season. The original sexual character of these biological phenomena gradually disappears as they become organically fixed and achieve functional independence. Although there can be no doubt that music originally belonged to the reproductive sphere, it would be an unjustified and fantastic generalization to put music in the same category as sex. Such a view would be tantamount to treating of Cologne Ca-thedral in a text-book of mineralogy, on the ground that it consisted very largely of stones.
>
> (Jung 2014c: 136).

The important point I want to emphasise is Jung's notion that such expressions of libidinal drives can achieve 'functional independence' from their original role as biological sexual drives. Another term for this phenomenon is exaptation – that is the use of an evolutionary adaptation for purposes other than those that led to its initial selection (Gould and Vrba 1982). In terms of Jung's theory, libidinal affects and drives that first evolved for breeding and the protection of the young could be utilised in other domains such as music. This process is part of Jung's broader conception of incest and endogamous kinship libido – that is, affects that bind members of a small family or kin group together (Jung 1983: 62). Such affects can, according to Jung, be repurposed (or exapted) in other forms of sociality. For example, religious affiliation may be based on deeper 'archetypal intuitions' related to the bond between children and parents, which then become the basis of adult forms of religious sociality (Jung 2014c: 89).

Abigail Tucker, in her book on maternal genes and brain neurochemistry, discusses at length research suggesting that human sexual and social bonding utilises very ancient neurochemistry that originally evolved to facilitate mammalian nurturant behaviour and infant bonding. As she evocatively writes: 'Mother love is the planet's original romance' (Tucker 2022: 40). From this perspective, the ancient neurobiological systems that subserve maternal care were repurposed or exapted in adult social and sexual bonding – or in Jung's terminology achieved functional independence. Significantly, such ancient maternal nurturant neurochemicals, seem to also underpin social bonding in music and dance, a finding that illuminates the neurobiology of human ritual and artistic life (Dissanayake 2021). Importantly, while acknowledging that what we have come to know as music may have originally been an expression of the reproductive instinct, Jung argues that it would be reductive to reduce it those original functions – as the analogy with the Cologne Cathedral makes clear.

Evidence for the exaptation of ancient mammalian neurobiology in sexual psychology is based on research demonstrating that romantic and maternal love are subserved by the same neural mechanisms. In this research, similar neural regions, and the neurochemical oxytocin, were activated in both cases. Additionally, in terms of romantic attachment, there was reduced negative social assessment and increased positive assessment suggesting possible neurological mechanisms as to why 'love makes blind.' The researchers argue that such findings enable us to understand the neural basis of one of the most 'formidable instruments of evolution,' which makes 'the procreation of the species and its maintenance a deeply rewarding and pleasurable experience' (Bartels and Zeki 2004: 1164).

Primatologist Sarah Blaffer Hrdy has commented on these findings, highlighting the evolutionary priority of maternal neurochemistry and its exaptation in human sexuality. She describes the 'euphoria' produced by neurochemicals released during birth and that both the maternal and infant brain during breast feeding release what she calls 'peace and bonding' hormones which serve to promote intimacy. Such 'elixirs of contentment,' she argues, also underpin sexual love:

… maternal sensations have clear evolutionary priority in the pleasure sphere. Long before any woman found sexual foreplay or intercourse pleasurable, her ancestors were selected to respond positively to similar sensations produced by birth and suckling, because finding these activities pleasurable would help condition her in ways that kept her infant alive. It would be more nearly correct, then, to refer to the "afterglow" from climax as an ancient "maternal" rather than sexual response.

(Hrdy 2000: 137)

Jaak Panksepp has written extensively on the use of the same neurochemical system in various forms of human social bonding and nurturant behaviour, highlighting that the affective basis of social care, as well as control of oxytocin secretion, seems to be based in primary process subcortical brain regions (Panksepp 2004; Panksepp and Biven 2012). Importantly, it is not just in female sexuality and parenting that subcortical neurochemistry is involved. For example, oxytocin levels have been found to peak in males during orgasm (Murphy et al. 1987). Additionally, human fathers not only show reductions in testosterone but also a similar pattern of hormone concentration to human mothers when interacting with their newborn infants (Storey et al. 2000). As one group of researchers writes fathers and mothers 'activate similar neural systems when exposed to child stimuli' adding that the experience of fatherhood decreases 'testosterone and increases in oxytocin' levels, changes in male neurochemistry that may 'support sensitive caregiving' (Glasper et al. 2019). Significantly, the activation in males of similar brain circuits and hormones evident in maternal nurturing has been termed a 'muted' version of the maternal experience in males (Wynne-Edwards and Reburn 2000; Wynne-Edwards 2001).

Panksepp has suggested that such findings provide some support for Freud's thesis of a connection between infantile and adult sexuality – an approach I suggest can also be fruitfully applied to Jung. As Panksepp writes:

> The nurturant circuits in the mother's brain and care-soliciting circuits in infants are closely intermeshed with those that control sexuality in limbic areas of the brain. This confluence lends modest support to controversial and widely debated Freudian notions of infantile sexuality and the possible relations between maternal love and female sexuality. Nurturance circuits can lead to the rapid learning of maternal behaviors, which then become permanent parts of a mother's behavioral repertoire. Males can also learn nurturant behaviors, and it is intriguing that sexual activity can strengthen antiaggressive, care giving substrates in male brains. We are finally deciphering the ancient neurosymbolic processes that first led to nurturance and social attachments in the mammalian brain. This work has important implications for the biological sources of friendship and love, as well as for sociopathy and psychiatric disturbances of affective contact such as autism.
>
> (Panksepp 2004: 246)

For Jung, the anima and animus are archetypal and consequently have greater phylogenetic depth than, as well as operating independently of, the conscious personality. As he writes, the 'autonomy of the collective unconscious expresses itself in the figures of anima and animus,' an autonomous aspect of the brain that represents the 'foundation stones of the psychic structure, which in its totality exceeds the limits of consciousness' (Jung et al. 1953: 20). Given Jung argued archetypes are located in unconscious, phylogenetically ancient subcortical brain regions (Jung 1960: 270–1), the above findings lend some credence to the notion of an archaic feminised component of the human male unconscious.

Jungian scholars have long noted the indebtedness of Jung's thinking to Goethe (Bishop 2008, 2007) and particularly the descent to 'The Mothers' scene of *Faust* (Edinger 1990: 54–60). Is it possible that what Goethe intuited about of the feminine dimension of existence is actually based on an evolved biological reality? In his *Goethe, Nietzsche, and Wagner: Their Spinozan Epics of Love and Power*, T.K. Seung argues that it is. As he writes during Faust's experience of rebirth and descent to the realm of 'The Mothers,' he abandoned the 'cognitive mode of existence and embraced its affective mode' (Seung 2006: 49). Commenting on this section of the play, Seung writes that '[m]aternal instinct is the strongest blood tie that holds together a family' while also suggesting that '[p]aternal love is not any less caring than maternal love. Paternal care is the activation of the maternal principle in the father' (Seung 2006: 53, 117 and 36).

Seung suggests that as Faust abandons the cognitive mode for the affective mode, he 'recants his blinding egotism and gains the inner light of communal bonds' (Seung 2006: 117). I suggest that such communal bonds may be based on neurochemistry in the male brain that supports 'sensitive caregiving' – neurobiological substrates shared by both males and females of our species. As I have argued elsewhere in my analysis of Goethe and Jung's thought, such a 'muted' version of the feminine principle in the male psyche may be what Jung had in mind with his concept of the anima – that is a less differentiated feminine component of male psychology that lay in the unconscious due to the predominance of male genes structuring the conscious mind (Clark 2022: 318).

Reconsidering Eros and Logos: Biological Archetypes or Linguistic Constructs

I have already suggested how genes and libido are important for Jung's evolutionary thought and his conception of sex-based differences. These evolved differences between female and male psychology are also central to his theory of sexual attraction. In this sense, they are the ancient emotional systems that evolved to bring women and men together in order that they reproduce and create offspring. Such attraction is, as I have intimated above, extremely ancient predating the very recent emergence of humans by millions of years. It is important to emphasise that while sexual reproduction in other species has affinities with reproduction in humans, there are also numerous difference that distinguish humans from other mammals and primates. It is in this context that I explore Jung's conception of sexual attraction, which, having an ancient biological origin, is also unique in qualitative and psychological terms. As Jung writes:

> Every man carries within him the eternal image of woman, not the image of this or that particular woman, but a definite feminine image. This image is fundamentally unconscious, an hereditary factor of primordial origin engraved in the living organic system of the man, an imprint or "archetype" of all the ancestral experiences of the female, a deposit, as it were, of all the impressions ever

made by woman—in short, an inherited system of psychic adaptation. Even if no women existed, it would still be possible, at any given time, to deduce from this unconscious image exactly how a woman would have to be constituted psychically. The same is true of the woman: she too has her inborn image of man ... Since this image is unconscious, it is always unconsciously projected upon the person of the beloved, and is one of the chief reasons for passionate attraction or aversion.

(Jung and Adler 2014: 198)

For Jung, the anima does not emerge *de novo* as a man reaches sexual maturity. His theory is based on the notion of an elaboration or development of ontogenetically prior structures, which then form the affective substrate of adult sexual attraction. For example, the experience of woman in the form of the mother is the male child's first emotional attachment to a female; as he writes, the 'mother-imago' derives from 'the collective archetype of the anima, which is incarnated a new in every male child' (Jung 1953: 14). He also mentions the mother as the male child's 'first love' going on to link the relationship with the mother to adult sexual emotion:

... in the realm of his psyche there is an image not only of the mother but of the daughter, the sister, the beloved the heavenly goddess, and the chthonic Baubo. Every mother and every beloved is forced to become the carrier and embodiment of this omnipresent and ageless image, which corresponds to the deepest reality in a man.

(Jung 1953: 12–3)

This perspective also suggests that both the maternal relationship and that of adulthood sexuality are not merely personal but are archetypal in nature. In this sense, the son invests the relation with the mother with the genetically inherited emotions characteristic of our species. Consequently, there is an impersonal dimension to the relationship whereby emotions that evolved millions of years prior to our birth colour our relationships. It is for this reason that Jung interprets the relation between mother and son in mythological terms, for it is in myth that such archaic archetypal structures are so saliently manifest. As he writes: 'For, in the relationship now reigning between them, there is consummated the immemorial and most sacred archetype of the marriage of mother and son .... At this level the mother is both old and young, Demeter and Persephone, and the son is spouse and sleeping suckling rolled into one' (Jung 1953: 12). It is worth noting that highly social pair-bonded mammals exhibit a 'more "infantile" distribution of oxytocin receptors' (Panksepp 2004: 272), an observation which gives support to the notion that sexual bonding and attachment between mothers and infants are subserved by the same very ancient neurobiological substrates.

Jung used the terms Eros and Logos to describe both the different orientations characteristic of female and male psychology as well as the contrasexual element in the psyche of each sex. As he avers the 'animus corresponds to the paternal

Logos just as the anima corresponds to the maternal Eros.' But this duality is not to be thought of as a strict or delimiting definition. For example, Eros and Logos are merely 'conceptual aids to describe the fact that woman's consciousness is characterized more by the connective quality of Eros than by the discrimination and cognition associated with Logos. In men, Eros, the function of relationship, is usually less developed than Logos' (Jung 1953: 14).

It is clear here that Jung does not seek to impose these concepts in a reductive way onto people's experience but is content to highlight general tendencies. For example, he states that in men Eros is *usually* less developed than Logos – which implies that it is not always so. Stevens has argued that, far from this passage being an example of Jung's deployment of sexist stereotypes, it accurately expresses a valid generalisation about archaic archetypes 'that possesses *statistical validity*' (Stevens 2002: 228). Jung did not have at his disposal the large cross-cultural data sets on sex-based differences now available to researchers – but his intuitions do seem generally correct and are supported by population level statistical trends. Additionally, while males do on average exhibit qualities that we might associate with Logos, and females with Eros, there is significant overlap between the sexes, particularly in cases where individuals identify with the social roles and behaviours of the opposite sex, an identification which frequently correlates with same-sex attraction (Vasey, Pocock, and VanderLaan 2007; VanderLaan, Ren, and Vasey 2013). These issues will be dealt with in more detail below where I discuss both the differences and similarities in male and female psychology and social behaviour and how such research enables us to see the underlying validity of many of Jung's claims regarding evolved sex-based differences.

It is important to emphasise that Jung saw the father as a crucial attachment figure for females, with her contrasexual animus being involved in this primary relationship as well as adulthood sexuality; as he writes '… as the mother seems to be the first carrier of the projection-making factor for the son, so is the father for the daughter' (Jung 1953: 14). When the contrasexual archetypes are activated, the experience of falling in love can seem unique and highly individualised; yet paradoxically, the pair is enacting an age-old archetypal experience:

This singular fact is due to the following circumstance: when animus and anima meet, the animus draws his sword of power and the anima ejects her poison of illusion and seduction. The outcome need not always be negative, since the two are equally likely to fall in love (a special instance of love at first sight). The language of love is of astonishing uniformity, using the well-worn formulas with the utmost devotion and fidelity, so that once again the two partners find themselves in a banal collective situation. Yet they live in the illusion that they are related to one another in a most individual way. In both its positive and its negative aspects, the anima/animus relationship is always full of "animosity" i.e., it is emotional and hence collective. Affects lower the level of the relationship and bring it closer to the common instinctual basis, which no longer has anything individual about it. Very often the relationship runs its course heedless of its human performers, who afterwards do not know what happened to them.

(Jung 1953: 11)

Jung goes on to contrast the experience of falling in love with the everyday routines of life:

What, after all, has commonplace reality to offer, with its registry offices, pay envelopes, and monthly rent, that could outweigh the mystic awe of the hieros gamos? ... The imperfections of real life, with its laborious adaptations and manifold disappointments, naturally cannot compete with such a state of indescribable fulfilment.

(Jung 1953: 12)

It was noted above that the neurobiological factors underpinning romantic love result in reduced avoidance behaviour and negative social assessment, with an increase in positive assessment and the triggering of reward mechanisms in the brain. Additionally, Hrdy described the neurochemicals involved in maternal attachment as 'elixirs of contentment' that give rise to a sense of 'peace and bonding.' These same mechanisms, she suggested, underpin sexual love and the associated subjective states – what Jung referred to as a state of 'indescribable fulfilment.'

It is important to note that the modern understanding of the role neurochemicals play in modulating emotion only became widely accepted in the second half of the twentieth century (Nichols 2013). Jung was near the end of his life when this revolution in psychology occurred, and he shows little evidence of adopting such perspectives in his later works. Additionally, much of the research cited in this book has only been undertaken in the last 30 years or so. We will never know what Jung would have made of this research. I suspect that he would have embraced it particularly as it seems to confirm some of his most basic intuitions. While I do not wish to reduce the phenomenology of such experiences to mere neurochemical mechanisms, it is clear that our most intimate emotional states are in fact chemically modulated. And it is such ancient neurochemistry that gives rise to the powerful emotions involved in sexual love – emotions that as Jung observes produce 'a state of indescribable fulfilment.'

Jung's ideas on the anima and animus have been subject to serious critique. For example, it has been argued that Jung's thinking on these issues derives from the confusion between archetype and cultural stereotype (Douglas 2000: 137). Additionally, it has been suggested that while Jung was astute in his analysis of the male unconscious and the pitfalls of projection, it seems that he may have at times not heeded his own warning and confused his anima projections with actual women (Nagy 1981: 66; Perera 1981: 40; Wehr 1987: 104; Douglas 2000: 34–51). Even if this is the case, however, it does not follow that his thinking on evolved biologically based sex differences is entirely illegitimate. That is, in the absence of such projections, the concepts of Eros and Logos still capture population level and cross-cultural trends in sex-based differences in social roles, psychology and behaviour.

It has also been argued that Jung's theory of sex-based differences is a product of Enlightenment binary thinking and a form of retrograde and politically conservative ideology that utilises biology and science to buttress its claims (Rowland 2002, 2004; Gardner and Gray 2016; Samuels 2016). These critiques represent a form of revisionism that seeks to reconfigure Jungian psychology so that it is more in accord with specific ideological and intellectual commitments. That is, the above authors seek to refashion analytical psychology in their own image – while rejecting Jung's explicitly stated position on evolved sex-based differences. However, there is another strand in Jungian scholarship that treats his theory of biologically evolved sex-based differences as foundational concepts in analytical psychology (Ulanov 1971, 1981; Neumann 1994; Stevens 2002). This latter group is more in accord with Jung's actual writing on the topic, whereas the former seeks to revise Jung's thinking on evolved sex-based differences.

For example, Samuels rejects Jung's concepts of Eros and Logos for their supposed problematic ideological implications (Samuels 2016). As Samuels elaborates, Jung delineates 'eros as an archetypal principle of psychological functioning' involving 'connectedness, relatedness [and] harmony' and the association of 'logos' with the masculine principles of 'rationality, logic, intellect [and] achievement' (Samuels 2016: 188). Samuel's objection to these aspects of Jung's thinking is based on the assumption that any psychological differences between the sexes that are biologically based and manifestations of evolved bodily and anatomical differences are inherently problematic in terms of contemporary sexual politics. As he writes:

> … the argument that innate psychological differences between the sexes are based on the body has serious and insidious difficulties in it. It *sounds* so grounded, so reasonable, so common-sensical, so different from social or ideological styles of exploring gender issues. However, if psychological activity is body-based then, as body is more or less a constant over the entire history of humanity, body-based psychological theory can only *support* the horrendous gender situation with which we are faced just now. For, if it is body-based, how can it be altered?
>
> (Samuels 2016: 101)

Samuels is correct to observe that the body is more or less constant throughout history – I would add over hundreds of thousands if not millions of years, as the basic biological substrates upon which our psychology is based reach into the deep past. It is a *non-sequitur* however to infer from this constancy that biologically based theory supports a 'horrendous gender situation.' For example, numerous feminists base their critiques of sex-based violence on the assumption of evolved sexual dimorphism in our species (Gowaty 1992, 2012; Hrdy 2000; Sullivan and Todd 2023; Phoenix 2023; Stock 2023). From this perspective, acknowledging biology is what enables us to understand the 'horrendous gender situation' and by understanding it, if not ameliorate it, then at least mitigate its most harmful and socially destructive effects.

Samuels is essentiality arguing for a form of dualism; that is, regardless of what bodies we possess, our psyche is separate from such embodied existence. Developing such a dualistic disembodied conception of the psyche he argues that the '... fact that a penis penetrates and a womb contains tells us absolutely nothing about the psychological qualities of those who actually possess such organs' (Samuels 2016: 101). In actual fact, the possession of a womb or a penis tells a great deal about the psychological qualities of the humans who possess them. The penis is the organ that ejaculates male genetic material in the form of sperm, which then fertilises the female ovaries. Those ovaries then gestate in the womb for nine months resulting in the birth of offspring. Throughout the animal kingdom, and among humans (for we are part of that kingdom), it is the fundamental differences in male and female reproductive biology that produce downstream differences in morphology, neurochemical regulation, and psychology. Our psychology is a product of our bodies and the associated reproductive strategies of each sex.

In their critique of Judith Butler's *Gender Trouble* (Butler 2011) and the academic discipline of gender identity theory, Sullivan and Todd have stated that 'gender identity theorists appear to believe that acknowledging biological differences between the sexes causes inequality.' They go on to argue that 'acknowledging sex differences is not the same as arguing that such difference justifies social and political inequality' (Sullivan and Todd 2023: 7). Countering the notion that the acknowledgement of sex differences entails a specific political ideology they write that the view 'that sex matters does not reflect a belief in a particular theory or creed. It is an unassailable fact' (Sullivan and Todd 2023: 5).

This view is shared by feminists who argue that the belief in biological differences between the sexes, far from being a construct that creates oppression, is actually a necessary prerequisite for understanding it and working towards its amelioration (Gowaty 1992, 2003; Hrdy 2000; Gowaty 2012). As evolutionary biologist Patricia Gowaty writes when reflecting on the need for a reproachment between feminism and the evolutionary sciences:

> Feminism and evolutionary biology are inextricably linked along many edges. Feminists building critiques of the rules of social life that place women in subordinate positions to men and as objects of sexist oppression are confronted with questions about the nature of women and men. Thus, feminist theorists implicitly develop theories of human nature ... which I think could be aided - explicitly and implicitly - by knowledge of the diversity of the biotic world and use of the comparative method, some of which can be supplied by evolutionary biologists. Theories of human nature developed by evolutionary biologists can likewise be aided by a feminist standpoint.
>
> (Gowaty 1992)

Some of the concerns Gowaty raises from an evolutionary point of view are control of female reproduction, sexual coercion and rape (Gowaty 1992). Primatologist Sarah Blaffer Hrdy has stated that female libido and sexual assertiveness 'are dangerous predispositions' that in many parts of the world are 'likely to get a woman beaten, disfigured, or killed' (Hrdy 2000: 223). She also argues that there is a 'widespread misconception that "biology is destiny" … According to this view if even a portion of the human male's dominance is ascribed to evolutionary causes, an intolerable status quo will have to be condoned as fundamentally unalterable' (Hrdy 1999: 2). These forms of oppression impact millions of women worldwide and the fundamental reason for that oppression is their underlying biology related to sexuality and reproduction. For example, cross-cultural data indicate that men commit up to 90 per cent of homicides, with women suffering high rates of sexual and domestic violence globally (Daly and Wilson 1990; Cepeda, Lacalle-Calderon, and Torralba 2022). Such violence is generally not a characteristic of the female sex. This is one reason among many why biological sex matters.

This is the case across primate species where males, due to their larger size and greater strength, frequently dominate females. However, here is the important point: female primates, including human females, seem to have evolved strategies that can protect them against males, and mitigate the threat they and their offspring may face (Buss 2021). It is important to emphasise that acknowledging evolved sex differences are important for understanding violence against women does not entail the position that male violence is biologically determined. There are also important sociocultural variables involved. But statistically and cross-culturally, men are the sex that commit violent crime, and women are often their victims (Buss 2021). It is this sexual asymmetry that may have driven certain adaptations in women – for example, the formation of kin-based coalitions that can provide safety and protection from potential threats (Power 2022a). It may even be the case that such coalitions ended up changing the trajectory of male behaviour and psychology over evolutionary time – as I explore in more detail below.

Samuel's main concern is with inferences from bodily differences to psychological differences, and that such psychological differences are believed to biologically determined – or in his words that 'anatomy is destiny.' As he writes, if 'anatomy is destiny, then nothing can be done to change the position of women. So women who base their quest for a new and positive meaning for femininity on the body inadvertently undermine their own cause' (Samuels 2016: 103). This position is in contrast to Hrdy's noted above where she called the notion that 'biology is destiny' a 'widespread misconception' (Hrdy 1999: 2). Darwinian feminists like Hrdy and Gowaty believe that biological differences play a very important role in human social life – but such differences, however important they may be, are only one variable among many others of a more sociocultural nature. Acknowledging evolved sex differences by no means entails the belief that biology is destiny in any rigid and deterministic manner.

Samuel's position is political and not necessarily scientific, although he does draw on studies that purportedly support his own social constructionist assumptions while rejecting scientific findings that undermine those assumptions. Such a critique is based on Samuel's somewhat dubious conflation of 'sex-specific psychologies' with right wing political ideology (Samuels 2016: 105). It is important to note that these are not the same thing and while conservatives may use biological differences between the sexes to buttress their ideological outlook, such an outlook does not create such differences, which exist prior to the cultural meanings attributed to them. As I noted above the view 'that sex matters does not reflect a belief in a particular theory or creed. It is an unassailable fact' (Sullivan and Todd 2023: 5). Samuels makes his position clear on this issue when he writes that 'I am sure that anatomy is not destiny and am trying to work my resentment at the idea that it might be into a critique of those who tell me it is. There are no *direct* messages from the body' (Samuels 2016: 103).

Samuel's is not wrong to be sceptical of the ideological uses to which anatomical and sex-based differences in psychology may be ideologically framed and deployed. Yet it is one thing to critique the manner in which sex-based differences are constructed and inscribed with cultural meanings; it is quite another to make the further inference that because of such inscription such differences do not exist and are entirely an artefact of cultural and ideological construction. As I will argue below, the kind of dualism and negation of bodily and the associated psychological differences, argued for by Samuels, finds very little support from the vast literature in neuroscience, cognitive psychology, anthropology, primatology and evolutionary studies.

Rowland, building on the work of Judith Butler, Jaques Derrida, Hauke and Samuels (Hauke 2000; Butler 2011; Derrida 2016) has also questioned the utility of Jung's concept of Eros and Logos from the perspective of poststructuralism and postmodern critiques of linguistic binaries (Rowland 2002, 2004). Like Samuels she doubts the validity of these concepts because of their putative ideological implications, what she refers to as politically conservative positions on innate 'feminine nature' (Rowland 2002: 48). Her revisionist approach to Jung consequently seeks to align his thinking with what she perceives to be contemporary political sensibilities. As she writes her approach seeks to 'explore the gender politics' of Jung's work and to 'offer a feminist revision that would look at his place in the gender politics of knowledge in the modern world' (Rowland 2002: vii). Further, in her feminist deconstructive approach, Rowland argues that the concepts Eros and Logos are an expression of Jung's binary and oppositional thinking derived from the Enlightenment. As she avers:

In his drive to grand theory, he desires to connect with and to imitate Enlightenment grand narratives. Most significantly from a feminist point of view, Jung is most deeply a man of the Enlightenment in his retention of oppositional thinking about gender. Indeed, gender becomes the principle means by which oppositional thinking is expressed in Jungian ideas. It is hard to imagine how the

essential deconstructive process of individuation could describe opposition between conscious and unconscious without Jung's typical use of gender.

(Rowland 2002: 139)

Consequently, Rowland concludes that the gendered binaries underpinning
Jung's Enlightenment outlook and the associated concepts of Eros and Logos have
'nothing to offer postmodern feminism' (Rowland 2002: 144). Rowland's charac-
terisation of Jung deploying 'oppositional thinking about gender' is inaccurate –
although it does enable her to obfuscate his actual theories by imposing on them a
poststructuralist analysis predicted on the putative prevalence of such oppositional
concepts in his work. It would be more correct to say that the poststructuralist theo-
rist constructs these concepts as oppositional, and then reads such oppositionality
into Jung's works. Which of course is very different from Jung's ideas being in and
of themselves oppositional. As I pointed out above, Jung's theories refer to archaic
archetypes that possess '*statistical validity*' (Stevens 2002: 228). A statistical trend
of this kind is a population level phenomenon in which different groups cluster into
a bimodal distribution, with each distribution having a different mean. Sex differences represent such a statistical phenomenon. An understanding of psychology
based on such bimodal and cross-cultural distributions of demographic data has
nothing to do with 'oppositional thinking' – for example, in a bimodal distribution
there is overlap between both groups, which means the groups are not 'oppositional' but actually have some shared tendencies despite the average differences.

The collection of essays, *Feminist Views From Somewhere: Post-Jungian
Themes in Feminist Theory*, also offers a critique of Jung's theories on sex-based
differences that like Samuels and Rowland sees such ideas as oppressive ideological constructs (Gardner and Gray 2016). One of the ideas explored in the volume is
that there is no neutral perspective from which we can think about issues of sex and
gender – that is, all attempts to develop an objective understanding of the psyche
are ultimately futile as all such attempts will always be 'existentially and socially
located' (Gardner and Gray 2016: xviii). The authors include in this category of
socially located discourses Jung's notion that the collective unconscious has an
'objective reality' independent of the observing mind as well as social categories
such as sex and gender. Regarding the latter they are particularly concerned with
Jung's 'antiquated and harmful ideas' about what it means to be 'female and his
creation of the rigid concepts of anima and animus' (Gardner and Gray 2016: xiv).
Gardner and Gray make a similar error to Rowland: a statistical trend is neither
oppositional nor is it rigid.

In developing their critique, Gardner and Gray use the example of a male geneti-
cist who epitomises the approach of evolutionary theory:

In his world, selection and survival are the *telos* of nature, of existing and being
in the world. Species select the best characteristics to ensure their survival in the
worlds in which they live. Sexual and natural selection determine species order.
Selection and survival are principally the concern of the male of the species ...

[Some scientists] might hold that peacocks grow beautiful tails to attract willing peahens so that the best progeny can be produced. The peahens blindly follow the seductive beauty of the peacock's tail, make no decisions and are passive rather than active in the procreative process.

(Gardner and Gray 2016: xvii)

The authors then go on to infer a lineage from Aristotle to modern genetics in which gendered constructs are imposed on the world: as they write 'the peacock and peahen example ... instantiates assumptions found in the philosophy of Aristotle – male/active, female/passive, the male provides the form, the female the matter of procreation.' Such a view they contend 'is embedded in a specific, gendered, view of the world' (Gardner and Gray 2016: xvii–xviii).

This ancient lineage of oppressive binary opposition is one that the modern male scientist unknowingly subscribes to and perpetuates – that is, he fails to 'locate his views in a specific, scientific, male culture that creates a perspective bias that has an immediate effect on the theory he espouses' (Gardner and Gray 2016: xvii). The authors reject an evolutionary approach to analytical psychology as they see such a conception as itself inherently gendered by a male orientation and that such a male-orientated science, and its broader cultural contexts, still serves to silence women in contemporary society; as they aver 'under the umbrella' of 'male' or 'neutral' theory or practice, women's 'voices are not listened to or heard by men as a whole social practice' and that consequently contemporary women's voices are still 'trivialized and discounted' (Gardner and Gray 2016: xviii). In essence, their critique asserts that from Aristotle to Jung and modern genetics and evolutionary theory, a gendered binary has been formulated by men to ensure women remain oppressed and silenced.

This critique is not without some merit. It is true that evolutionary theory was first developed by men and that such men unconsciously imbued their theories with patriarchal social attitudes and biases. Such biases are particularly evident in the works of nineteenth-century evolutionary theorists (Hrdy 2000: 10–26; Diogo 2024). This did result in an emphasis on male behaviours such as hunting or male mate choice – and the attendant neglect of the active role females play in evolutionary processes. However, evolutionary theory has progressed a great deal since then and particularly so in the last half-century. It is now a discipline that centres female perspectives and the important role that female strategies, alliances, friendships and mothering play in the social life of primates as well as our own species – and this revolutionary and innovative work has been undertaken predominantly by women (Lawick-Goodall 1968; Tanner and Zihlman 1976; Goodall 1986, 1996; Hrdy 1999, 2000, 2009; Hager 2005; Hawkes and Coxworth 2013; Smuts 2017). There is no evidence that contemporary evolutionary theory is a male-orientated science or that it silences the voices of women.

An alternative to the views articulated by Samuels, Rowland and Gardner and Gray can be found in the work of Ann Belford Ulanov, Erich Neumann and Sylvia Perera, all of whom adopt a biologically informed approach to analytical psychology (Perera 1981; Ulanov 1971, 1981; Neumann 1994). Ulanov has developed a theory of sexual polarity based on fundamental differences in male and female bodies and associated psychology. For her, the polarity of masculine and feminine, while grounded in ineluctable somatic differences, nevertheless becomes the basis for more malleable expressions of such polarity at the level of culture and its associated imagery. In this way, she manages to navigate a path between the Scylla and Charybdis of biology and cultural factors. As she writes when commenting on Jung's conception of the psyche, and how his theories may be reconceptualised in the context of modern debates regarding the role of culture in the formation of identity:

> To be without sexual distinctions would to be without psychical structure. Instead of the freedom that the representatives of the cultural school seek – from sexual roles that dictate styles of identity to men and women – Jung's view asserts that the denial of sexual differences would lead to a lack of structure that would prevent a person from achieving any identity at all. The structure of the psyche in various polarities is not simply a product of cultural influence, although, of course, the way that these polarities are conceived and evaluated is indeed subject to cultural forces. Thus Jung might argue the current challenges to sexual distinction by saying that the way we conceive of and value psychic polarities, which are symbolized most often in masculine-feminine terms, may vary according to cultural influence, but the fact of psychic polarities and the centrality of the masculine-feminine polarity is a basic structure of the human psyche.
>
> (Ulanov 1971: 145–6)

For Ulanov, cultural stereotypes as well as images of sexual polarity, are an outgrowth of more fundamental differences associated with sexed bodies. In this sense, it is inevitable that stereotypes of male and female develop as we mature form childhood and into adulthood, as such stereotypes are crucial in the process of identity formation and the growth of healthy sexuality. However, stereotypes associated with sexual polarity can all too easily become reified into rigid social roles that can be both socially and psychologically oppressive – both to those who promulgate them and to those who may be their victims. In this sense, the healthy differentiation of consciousness from the unconscious, in Ulanov's view, involves identity formation structured by sexual polarity. Yet as we mature, we become increasingly aware of the contrasexual principle within ourselves and the culture more generally. It is this assimilation of otherness that facilitates the growth and expansion of consciousness.

Of primary importance for Ulanov is that every human being is born from the body of a woman – as she writes we 'are born of women; we partake of female flesh; we emerge from female bodies which produce food and nourish us. Our mothers are the first to bond with us psychologically' (Ulanov 1981: 72–3). Additionally, as we mature, the experience of male and female is crucial to identity formation.

As she writes when commenting on the early formation of sexual polarity: 'In un-folding its young self a child quickly comes to acquire gender identity as male or female' (Ulanov 1981: 48). It is during this process of identity formation that stere-otypes may be useful in distinguishing self from other; however, in Ulanov's view, this process may differ in boys and girls, given that boys separate from the femi-nine as they mature, whereas girls remain part of the feminine domain:

> In growing up both consciously and unconsciously we gather loosely defined images of the feminine from our experiences of women, our perception of their behaviour, our feelings about them ... Boys seeking a masculine self-image, initially project this feminine content onto all the females they meet, thereby demarking the male's psychological territory from the female's. The boy's dif-ficulty in making his first claims to identity centre on seeing himself as separate from the mother, the original harbour of being, that authority of body and soul. The girl's difficulty in securing her own identity as female centres on finding her own place within the identification with her mother, a likeness which does not swallow up her distinct individuality.
>
> (Ulanov 1981: 59)

As we become adults, a similar process of projection occurs as we mature sexu-ally; as Ulanov avers in 'sexual matters projection helps us distinguish between things masculine and feminine ... the intimacies of sexual love open deeper expe-riences of finding oneself in the loving embrace of the other, who is insufficiently different to mark off the boundaries of self and sufficiently alike to reinforce com-mon humanness' (Ulanov 1981: 48). Significantly, Ulanov links adult sexuality with the bond between mother and infant writing that only an 'adult sexuality in a true love relationship can match the mother-infant relationship ... As a mother mir-rors the face of her child, so a lover reflects the face of the beloved' (Ulanov 1981: 48). This view echoes research discussed above about the shared neurobiological substrates evident between mother and infant attachment and sexual bonding.

It is in this process of development from childhood to full adult maturity where the potential danger lurks if sexual polarity is reified into rigid categories; as she writes, the existence in society of 'reified, prescriptive sexual stereotyping pre-supposes an antecedent radical splitting up of that central and early perception of otherness which is inherent in sexual polarity' (Ulanov 1981: 34–35). And while stereotypes may initially facilitate distinctions between masculine and feminine, if they are reified into rigid social roles in such a manner they may 'eventually cripple awareness.' Linking the psychological with the social, Ulanov argues that the pro-jection of stereotypes on to others in a rigid manner 'almost inevitably fuels social oppression' (Ulanov 1981: 60).

While Ulanov is critical of the emergence of rigid stereotypes out of a more pri-mary situation of sexual polarity, as intimated above, she is also critical of attempts to deny such polarity. In her view, the denial of these primary differences can also thwart the process of conscious differentiation from the unconscious. And such lack of differentiation can give rise to both personal and socio-political dysfunctions:

> Repressing sexual polarity amounts to denying the evidence of our senses, of body differences, and of the reception of the psychological significance of those differences. To repress this knowledge requires huge expenditure of energy that builds up enormous tensions in the unconscious. This sets the stage for the inevitable return of the repressed content by devious routes, usually in heightened agitation about almost all other polarities, as if conscripting them to play the central symbolic role that sexual symbolism so long enjoyed.
>
> (Ulanov 1981: 40)

By denying the embodied nature of sexual polarity, and the manner in which it structures the unconscious, the human personality, according to Ulanov, is thwarted in the task of achieving wholeness, which requires conscious awareness and integration of those unconscious processes. This situation gives rise to a new set of abstractions and consciously formulated polarities that, similar to the process of stereotype reification, maintains a condition of dissociation from the unconscious. As she writes, 'displacement of sexual polarization onto political polarisation' may be expressed in the 'dualism of oppressor and oppressed.' In this sense, sexual polarity is believed to have been formulated as a system of oppressive stereotypes and that consequently in order to be liberated from such oppression such polarity must be undermined and rejected. In this situation 'sexual stereotypes are transmogrified into rigidly prescriptive roles for political activists' – which in the most extreme case justify rage and violence based on a 'polarity of "us" (the oppressed) and "them" (the oppressor)' (Ulanov 1981: 40).

Ulanov is not opposing movements for political liberation nor the liberation of women. Her point is that, given differences between the sexes have historically been linked with the oppression of women some 'see the only solution to that injustice in the abolition of sexual differences entirely.' In her view this denial of differences between the sexes 'would simply add psychological injustice to social injustice.' Consequently, she argues that discrimination 'against women must of course be ended, but repression of sexual differences will not achieve that end' (Ulanov 1971: 175). This view is very much in accord with the authors discussed above who base their analysis of female oppression, and its potential amelioration, in a biologically grounded conception of sexual dimorphism (Gowaty 1992, 2012; Hrdy 2000; Sullivan and Todd 2023; Phoenix 2023; Stock 2023).

Ulanov's point is that such liberation should be grounded in an awareness of sexual polarity for the historical oppression of women was, in her view, predicted on the psychosocial oppression of the feminine principle within the human psyche – both at the personal and collective levels. It follows from this assumption that a liberatory political programme needs to address the oppression of the feminine dimension of life. The error, in the social constructionist view according to Ulanov, resides in the assertion that feminine imagery is an artefact of an oppressive social system – oppression that is both encoded in and enforced by language.

It is for this reason that Ulanov rejects the notion that the putatively oppressive nature of sexual polarity is evident in the structure of language itself. Consequently she also rejects the notion that changing language can form the basis of political change. As she writes a 'change in grammar is not an adequate response to the exclusion of women and of the feminine in collective consciousness' (Ulanov 1981: 51). Here, we can see in her work an implicit critique of theories, such as those proposed by Rowland and Derrida, that postulate binaries are created by language as opposed to being described by language. For Ulanov, sexual polarity is deeper and more primary than language. Evolutionary science would suggest this approach is correct as the binary of male and female evolved millions of years prior to the emergence of hominins – further within the hominin lineage the binary of male and female existed long before we evolved the linguistic capacity to describe sexual polarity.

Erich Neumann has outlined a developmental approach to sex-based differences similar to Ulanov's. Neumann's approach is grounded in anthropology as well as an acknowledgement of the importance of female reproductive cycles to the symbolic aspects of cultural development. Significantly, unlike the work of Samuels and Rowland, Neumann's approach is consilient with modern research in evolutionary anthropology. For example, Neumann focusses on the intergenerational alliances that women form with support networks with older women being of prime importance. In the following quote, the influence of Bachofen and Briffault, and the theory of matrilineal social organisation discussed in Chapter 1, is clear:

> It is typical for the phase of Self-conservation that psychologically and often sociologically the woman remains in the women's group – the mother clan – and maintains her continuity "upward" in relationship to the group of mothers and "downward" to the group of daughters. Her solidarity with the proximity to women and the Feminine coincide with her segregation and sense of alienation from men and the masculine.
>
> (Neumann 1994: 11)

This is a widely reported phenomenon in both primates and hunter-gatherer cultures (Whiting et al. 1988; Kramer 2005; Benenson 2019). As they grow, young girls tend to congregate closer to the camp where other women are caring for and raising children more than young boys do, who tend to range further from the camp. Evolutionary anthropologists have argued that this tendency to congregate around the women's camp enables young girls to not only assist in childcare as part of a matrilineal alloparenting system, but to also benefit themselves from such early experiences. For example, the offspring of girls who do have such early experience in childrearing seem to have higher rates of survival – and the absence of such experience may adversely impact offspring. This preference of young and adolescent girls to seek out infants and young children to care for may be an adaption for parenting – of learning how to mother. Given it exists not only in humans, but numerous primate species, it is most likely a very ancient aspect of human sex-based social psychology (Maestripieri and Pelka 2002; Edwards 2002; Hrdy 2009: 217–9). This tendency of girls to stay closer to the mother and maternal domain, due to being the same sex as the mother, with boys tending to separate, was also noted above by Ulanov (Ulanov 1981: 59).

Neumann consequently sees male and female development to be different in significant ways. And these differences, as modern research suggests, is most likely associated with different developmental and hormonal profiles in males and females:

> The physical changes from infant to boy, youth, man, and greybeard, are also accompanied by psychic changes that differ greatly from the corresponding changes in the development of woman. Hence between the sexes we must assume a biopsychic difference that is manifested in archetypal and symbolic ways, even if it cannot be expressed in any strict characterological categories. Therefore the Self as the totality of the personality rightly carries secondary sexual characteristics, and both body and psyche are closely connected in their dependence on hormones.
>
> (Neumann 1994: 6–7)

Neumann has commented on the role of pubertal initiation rituals which seek to manage the transition from childhood, through adolescence and into adulthood. He noted that during this period of separation from the maternal domain, that young males can be particularly prone to hebephrenia, a subset of schizophrenia characterised by hallucinations and delusions that tends to afflict adolescents:

> In so-called primitive cultures rites of initiation under the protection of the rituals of the collective take place during puberty because this period of time is particularly significant but also dangerous; in such rites the youth is conclusively delivered from the maternal realm and inducted into the patriarchal. By contrast, in our culture, which possesses only remnants of these initiatory rites, this important "transitional phase"—on the way toward a strengthened masculinity and the initial attempts at coming to terms with sexuality, partner, and world—is stigmatized by an abundance of neurotic complaints, even by hebephrenia, an illness typically appearing at this time.
>
> (Neumann 1994: 250)

Among Indigenous groups in Australia, such initiation rites involve the separation of young boys from the community of women and children and integration into the 'intergenerational chain' of men and fathers. Importantly, it is at this time that the neophyte is first introduced to the sacred objects associated with his totem – for example, the *churingas* discussed in Chapter 2 (Munn 1984: 58). While the nature of such transitional rites differs among Indigenous groups, from initiating young boys into the community of male hunters, to solidarity among males who must organise for warfare, they all seem to share some level of hardship and endurance as the young boy transitions from the domain of his mother and the other women of the community, into the community of men (Lee 1979; Sosis, Kress, and Boster 2007: 235–40). Such a process of separation from the community of women does not characterise the ontogeny of female socio-cognitive development – in fact, young girls and women remain in that domain as Neumann pointed out above.

Neumann's conceptualisation of the feminine or Eros highlights a number of factors associated with the cycles in nature and the cycles of the body, factors which he juxtaposes with the masculine principle or Logos. His association between sexuality and the moon is part of a long tradition in Western culture from Aristotle to Shakespeare's *A Midsummer Night's Dream* where sexual energies are unleashed in a moon lit forest (Chiari 2018: 35). There is also the 'explicitly lunar attributes' of hunter's deities such as the Greek Artemis and the Roman Diana in addition to hunting ritual and folklore throughout much of the world that links moonlight, hunting and female reproductive cycles (Knight 1995: 38). These connections may have deep roots in the past given the association between female reproductive cycles and the moon in Indigenous cultures from Africa to South America and Australia (Lewis 2008; Knight and Lewis 2016; Casiraghi et al. 2021).

Neumann adopts a chronobiological conception of the psyche in which psychological and bodily changes are linked with natural cycles such as night and day and lunar cycles. Consequently, he emphasises the importance of the duality of nighttime sleep and daytime wakefulness, and specific associations between monthly female reproductive cycles and the moon. As he writes when commenting on the latter, the 'significance of the moon as chronometer stands in the foreground of the moon cult' adding that the 'moon guides primitive humankind's orientation in time' (Neumann 1994: 84). Neumann goes on to aver that new moon and full moon 'are the earliest sacred times.' In Neumann's view, female reproductive cycles were once linked to the 'moon's periodicity' although in contemporary women the 'inner lunar period has made itself independent of the external moon' (Neumann 1994: 85).

Neumann links attunement to lunar cycles with the matrilineal theory of human cultural evolution; as he writes 'moon-consciousness is matriarchal consciousness' (Neumann 1994: 84). He juxtaposes this form of 'qualitative' temporality which is 'rhythmical and periodic' with the 'abstract, quantitative time of … scientific, patriarchal consciousness' with its cold sense of 'objectivity' and abstraction which is 'more distanced from reality' (Neumann 1994: 84 and 87). Such patriarchal consciousness Neumann associates with the 'systematized mind' which he contrasts with his conception of matriarchal 'non-systematized, open consciousness' that is capable of being 'expanded' (Neumann 1994: 96 and 98). Neumann links the patriarchal orientation with the 'consciousness world of logos' which is associated with the male's greater 'degree of isolation but equally to the intensified formation and solidity of ego and consciousness' (Neumann 1994: 8). Neumann's association of systematising with male Logos is supported by modern experimental psychology indicating males on average have higher levels of systematising traits than females (Connellan et al. 2000; Baron-Cohen 2003, 2020; Ruigrok et al. 2014).

The duality between of Eros and Logos is also part of Neumann's theory of creativity, where dance, music, the unconscious and sleep are linked, with creativity in the male resulting from activation of the feminine contrasexual principle or anima. As he writes 'in their emphasis on rhythm, music and dance ... play a significant role for the attitude and the establishment of matriarchal consciousness' (Neumann 1994: 87). Additionally, the 'moon-spirit' is more easily activated 'during the night with its enlivenment of the unconscious and the attendant introversion than in the light of day' with sleep and its associated circadian rhythms having the power to regenerate 'the body and its wounds.' (Neumann 1994: 84 and 101). And in terms of creativity, Neumann in much the same manner as Jung, avers that 'the male artist, in whom the anima, his female side (and with the anima also the matriarchal consciousness), is more strongly accentuated than in the average patriarchal man' (Neumann 1994: 13). As he elaborates on these associations:

It is the regenerative power of the unconscious that does its work during sleep, in the darkness of the night or in the light of the moon, as a mystery and in mystery, from out of itself, from nature, without the influence of consciousness and without the help of the head-ego. This is why the healing pill and the healing plant are assigned to the moon, and their secret is protected and preserved by women, or better, by the Feminine, which belongs to the moon.

(Neumann 1994: 102)

In Neumann's conception, Eros represents the pole in the psyche associated with 'relatedness and relationship' which he juxtaposes with the systematising and abstracting impulse of Logos. The greater differentiation of Logos in male psychology results 'in a certain opposition to female psychology,' an opposition that has significant therapeutic relevance; as Neumann elaborates as an expression of 'fear of relationship, this fundamental experience lurks in the background of many neuroses in men.' Yet, this is not an entirely negative aspect of human psychology; for example 'masculine consciousness' underpins 'science and objectivity' with its 'conceptual world ... of abstraction' (Neumann 1994: 105 and 213). As he elaborates:

Patriarchal, archetypally masculine consciousness is a most significant and, as the development of *Homo sapiens* shows, exceedingly successful organ of adaptation and information processing. One of its advantages lies in its ongoing readiness to react, and in the extraordinary rapidity of its reaction and adaptation ... The rapidity of conscious reaction ... is increased by all those processes that have led to the freeing of patriarchal consciousness from the unconscious.

(Neumann 1994: 93)

It is important to note that Neumann is not attributing Eros and Logos to males and females as such for both principles are operative to different degrees in each sex. The point is the degree to which the principles of Eros and Logos are differentiated in each sex.

While the cultural associations Neumann is describing are widely known, is there scientific evidence of an evolutionary association between female reproductive biology and lunar cycles? There is abundant cross-cultural evidence of the association between women, menstruation and the moon which may have to do with various forms of periodicity and the linking of sexual politics to lunar cycles (Knight and Lewis 2016; Power 2017, 2022a). This association has been long acknowledged by Jungians (Harding 1936: 39–54; Neumann 1994: 64–119). Significantly, evidence from African foragers has demonstrated an association between hunting, ritual life and sexual politics, with these aspects of social life being linked to lunar cycles. In this sense, the connection is at the very least cultural – with possible biological roots in the deep past (Power 2022a). For example, among the Western Pygmy BaYaka, an African hunter-gatherer community, the linkage of menstrual taboos with the moon is explicit in the belief that 'women's biggest husband is the moon' (Lewis 2008: 299). However, while the lifecycles and evolved chronobiology of many animals follows lunar cycles, the evolutionary relationship between women's reproductive cycles and the moon is less clear (Kronfeld-Schor et al. 2013).

One of the problems researchers have found in linking human chronobiology to lunar cycles is that most modern humans live with artificial light, which interferes with how the body responds to natural fluctuations in light throughout the year. In order to address this issue, researchers compared two communities from South America that are culturally very similar but only one of which has access to electricity and hence artificial lighting. Significantly among these cultures, 'mythological stories associate the moon with the female reproductive cycle and sexual relations.' And like the example from Africa the moon is represented in these cultures as a man who has 'sexual relations with women' and who also induces the 'first menstruation and regulates the timing of the following menstruations' (Casiraghi et al. 2021: 5). Significantly, the researchers found on moonlit nights in the community without electricity that fishing, hunting, and social and sexual activities increased (Casiraghi et al. 2021). Some suggestive research has also found that women's menstrual cycles shortened and lost synchrony with exposure to artificial nocturnal light. Based on these findings, and the observation that many species synchronise reproductive behaviour with a particular phase of the lunar cycle in order to increase reproductive success, the authors speculate that 'in ancient times, human reproductive behavior was synchronous with the Moon' adding that our modern lifestyles have changed 'reproductive physiology and behavior' (Helfrich-Förster et al. 2021: 1).

The above discussion provides an outline of possible avenues of future research linking human chronobiology, culture and lunar cycles to various strands in the analytical psychology literature. It could be explored further in a more detailed analysis of Neumann's ideas in, for example, *The Great Mother: An Analysis of an Archetype*, as well critiques of his work by the archaeologist Marija Gimbutas, who extended the ideas of Jung and Neumann in her analysis of pre-Indo-European archaeological strata in Europe, which she believed lacked many of the features of later patrilineal cultures analysed in Neumann's earlier work (Gimbutas 2001: 316–20; Clark 2020: 149–53). Contemporary scientific research into associations between chronobiology and lunar cycles could also be explored in a reconsideration of Ester Hardings' classic Jungian analysis of the topic in *Woman's Mysteries: Ancient and Modern* (Harding 1936). In what follows, I explore such an interdisciplinary approach through a discussion of the work of Sylvia Perera. It is hoped that such ideas can be explored further by other researchers, particularly in the context of improving understanding of human chronobiology in the scientific community.

Sylvia Perera has built on the work of Neumann, Harding and others in her *Descent to the Goddess: A Way of Initiation for Women*. Perera's approach can be distinguished from those advanced by Rowland, Samuels and Gardner and Gray discussed above. The main difference is that Perera bases her theory on an understanding of neurobiology and female reproductive cycles. Like Ulanov she acknowledges women's unique biology and psychology yet argues that such uniqueness does not justify misogyny and oppression – rather, biology illuminates such oppression.

One of the issues Perera raises is the severing or suppression of a deep affective relationship between mothers and daughters. Importantly, as noted in Chapter 2 in my discussion of endogamy and ancient kinship and breeding systems, the relationship between daughters and their mothers (that is the grandmother of her children) is believed to be crucial to the evolution of our species. For example, grandmothers are believed to have provided much of the metabolic and social support necessary for the increase in brain and body size and associated with extension of ontogeny in the hominin lineage, possibly beginning some 2 million years go with the emergence of *Homo erectus* (O'Connell, Hawkes, and Blurton Jones 1999; Hrdy 2009; Hawkes and Coxworth 2013). Perera suggests such severing results from the suppression of the feminine in the broader culture – which manifests itself in suppression of the affective richness between mothers and daughters; as she writes '… too many modern women have not been nurtured by the mother in the first place' and have grown up in patriarchal familial and social contexts of 'abstract, collective authority.' The consequent identification with the father and with patriarchal culture, may result in alienation from the 'feminine ground and the personal mother, whom they have often seen as weak or irrelevant' (Perera 1981: 7).

Perera develops an historical and therapeutic conception of the feminine and masculine grounded in a broader theory of ritual descent. This model builds on the ancient Sumerian myth of the descent of Innana, which Perera interprets in terms of a descent into primary process neurobiological systems involving sacrifice of secondary process ego consciousness. Such primary process systems consist of '[l]ower brain activities that regulate peristalsis, menstruation, pregnancy, and other forms of bodily life to which we must submit' (Perera 1981: 24). She also associates such primary process systems with 'the psychology of creativity and the early, pre-oedipal stages of human development and their pathologies' arguing that such descent involves a 'sacrifice of the upper-world aspects of the Self ... for the sake of the dark, different, or altered-state aspects.' Such a transition from second-ary process forms of ego consciousnesses into primary process altered states repre-sents a descent to the 'repressed, undifferentiated ground of being with the hope of gaining rebirth with a deeper, resonant awareness' (Perera 1981: 14).

However, such descent is not without its dangers for both patient and therapist:

> These deepest descents lead to radical reorganization and transformation of the conscious personality. But, like the shaman's journey or Inanna's, they are fraught with real peril. Hopefully in therapy the therapist may "manage" and companion the descents with help from the unconscious, but some fall beyond the therapist's capacity or open into the unseen crevasses of psychotic episodes. All descents provide entry into different levels of consciousness and can en-hance life creatively. All of them imply suffering. All of them can serve as initia-tions. Meditation and dreaming and active imagination are modes of descent. So too are depressions, anxiety attacks, and experiences with hallucinogenic drugs.
>
> (Perera 1981: 50)

It is important in this context to note that dreams, psychosis, altered states, mys-tical or spiritual experiences, all seem to involve reversions to primary process styles of thinking (Hobson 1999; Hobson, Hong, and Friston 2014; Hobson 2014). Additionally, archetypal themes are often experienced in such states due to the in-gestion of psychedelic hallucinogens (Carhart-Harris et al. 2014: 14; Clark 2021). This neuroscientific research confirms some of Perera's basic insights.

The additional value of Perera's approach is her suggestion that the transition to primary process modes of cognition during altered states, may have a unique quality for females due to the distinct biology associated with lower brain activities that regulate 'peristalsis, menstruation, pregnancy' (Perera 1981: 24). The different qualitative nature of female versus male altered states is worthy of further consid-eration – and Perera's work provides some very interesting suggestions as to how this could be undertaken in the context of the contemporary neuroscientific study of altered states of consciousness.

Perera associates the experience of *participation mystique* in altered states of consciousness and the associated preverbal, affect-based primary process systems with archaic matriarchal levels of awareness (Perera 1981: 59, 68 and 14). While she contrasts this mode with the abstract left brain conceptual discriminations of Apollonian Logos (Perera 1981: 12, 60, 30 and 24), the descent to primary process modes of being is not conceived of as a regressive abdication of styles of cognition associated with patriarchal Logos; on the contrary the material encountered in such descents can become objects of knowledge and integrated with the Logos functions of consciousness. In Perera's view, such knowledge requires us to go deep to re-claim modes of consciousness which are different from the intellectual, 'secondary process' levels the West has so well refined. However, knowledge gained from such descents, in Perera's view, needs to be integrated into the 'mental-cerebral, ordinary Western consciousness, in order to forge what Jean Gebser calls integral consciousness' (Perera 1981: 14).

In the above discussion, I have explored various aspects of human chronobiology and associations between female reproductively biology and natural cycles. In the anthropological literature these factors are often linked to aspects of male social life such as hunting, with menstrual blood and the blood of the hunt both being considered sacred and taboo. These two domains of life seem to operate in a dynamic sexual economy. Additionally, such associations are recurrent motifs cross-culturally. Given their ubiquitous presence, what are the possible evolutionary explanations for such phenomena?

I have already explored the model developed by Chris Knight and colleagues in Chapter 2. This thesis states that in our evolutionary past, coalitions of women were able to resist forms of male dominance by encouraging men to redirect reproductive and hunting effort into socially productive avenues. Blood became an important aspect of such group solidarity as Power writes when commenting on the ethnographic evidence of such social practices: 'women use idioms of bleeding together to express connection and belonging' (Power 2022a: 10). As already noted, this association of blood, hunting and female reproductive cycles is a common feature of hunter-gatherer societies globally (Knight 1988; Knight and Lewis 2016)

In Knight's model, in the distant evolutionary past, women would collectively withhold sex and then allow it, a pattern that oscillated with lunar cycles and male hunting effort. As Knight elaborates:

> It may make better Darwinian sense (and so begin to feel logical and emotionally satisfying) for males to nurture their own babies – hence their own genetic future – by acknowledging female solidarity, respecting its message, co-operating in the hunt and bringing back game to camp.
>
> (Knight and Lewis 2016: 95)

I noted above the upregulation of oxytocin in the male brain, and its association with prosociality, sexual bonding and male infant care. Knight's theory provides a possible explanation as to how this may have occurred: through female sexual selection males who were willing to share the bounty of the hunt would be preferred as mates and be at an evolutionary advantage relative to males who were unwilling to do so. In this model, it was female coalitions and female sexual selection that was the major driver of human evolutionary change. In Jungian terms, it was such female coalitions performing rituals in synchrony with lunar cycles that resulted in the evolution of the anima in the male brain – that is a more prosocial and feminine approach to parenting and social care.

In her paper 'The politics of Eros: ritual dialogue and egalitarianism in three Central African hunter-gatherer societies,' anthropologist Morna Finnegan elaborates on Knight's model in an exploration of African women's song, dance and ritual.

Her conception of Eros, the body and biology is antithetical to that proposed by Samuels, Rowland and Gardner. However, it provides some ethnographic support for the ideas developed by Ulanov, Neumann, Harding and Perera. This may be because the latter authors developed their theories based on a broader historical, mythological and anthropological analysis, whereas the former's theories represent a specifically Western theoretical and ideological conception of the human body, biology and sex.

Finnegan focusses on sexual politics and the important role the sexed body plays in the ritual life of egalitarian hunter-gatherers in Central Africa. While the culture of contemporary hunter-gatherers would differ in many ways from that of our archaic ancestors, they nevertheless do provide insights into the kinds of social organisation, sexual politics and ritual life that may have characterised humans prior to the advent of agriculture, hierarchised city states and modern industrial societies.

In justifying her use of the term Eros in the analysis of African hunter-gatherer ritual, Finnegan argues that the concept faithfully reflects the embodied nature of sexual politics in these cultures. As she writes, 'Eros classically indicated qualities such as love, lust, joy [and] intercourse.' Significantly, she quotes Freud's use of the term to describe libidinal instinct; as Freud writes 'the libidinal, sexual or life instincts ... are best comprised under the name of *Eros*' (Freud, Strachey, and Freud 2001: 258; Finnegan 2013: 700). The ritual dances that Finnegan analyses involve coalitions of women that foreground female sexuality and procreative capacity. Yet making female biology such a salient factor in these cultural practices by no means diminishes female political power; on the contrary it is biological difference that becomes the basis of female political assertion and autonomy. It is in this sense that the 'politics of Eros' is an apt way of conceptualising these forms of ritual life.

In discussing Judith Butler's *Gender Trouble* (Butler 2011), Finnegan contrasts the conception of sex advanced in gender theory with how it is often understood in the ethnographic literature. As she avers, there is 'an odd discordance in the reading of Western gender theory alongside ethnography of Central African hunter-gatherers. The two don't sit comfortably.' More specifically, Butler's conception of gender 'tends to hover unconvincingly above empirical data that stays rooted in sexed bodies and their metaphors.' In commenting on the influence of gender theory within some areas of anthropology, she states that it has become 'standard practice within feminist anthropology to repudiate any essential relationship between the biological body and cultural identity' – a perspective in which 'the ongoing deconstruction of the body has come to seem the only "natural" fact' (Finnegan 2013: 697).

For Finnegan African women's rituals foreground the 'visceral, libidinal power of the body in motion.' It is this focus on embodied sex that distinguishes her own ethnographic orientation from that of gender theorists; as she writes, anthropologists engaged in field work with African societies frequently comment on the 'symbolic preoccupation with the very terms recent Western gender theory disposes of at the outset – sex, menstrual blood, gestation, birth, and parturition' (Finnegan 2013: 697). As she writes:

> In its creativity and doubling capacity the body, particularly the female body, is a powerful cultural player. In a direct reversal of much Western philosophical and feminist theory, where biology is what diminishes or reduces the social person, biology here is what enlarges it … That the female procreative body could express a collective agency which is both active and political, an agency expressed through public ritual celebrations of reproductive sex, birth, blood, and the female genitals, has rarely been considered … [D]uring women's dances there is a recurrent statement about the specifically female power that is birth, and the sexual economy that runs parallel to it. In amplified body-statements, women publicly capitalize on their power as the producers of children.
>
> (Finnegan 2013: 707)

While some feminists, as well as Jungian scholars discussed in this chapter, do believe that 'biology is what diminishes or reduces the social person' it is not true that all feminist thought adopts such a view. For example, early feminists such as Mary Wollstonecraft (1759–1797), who were writing before contraception profoundly altered modern sexual politics, were fully aware of how biological asymmetries between the sexes negatively impacted women (Wollstonecraft and Brody 1992; Bachiochi 2021). At the heart of her analysis was the need for chastity as without it (both on the part of men and women) unintended pregnancies could occur – which impacts females more than males as females are the sex that gestates and gives birth to offspring. Wollstonecraft also sought greater rights for mothers and recognition of the importance of the domestic sphere for social life more generally. Wollstonecraft's ideas have been extended by a number of contemporary feminists who premise their ideas on the reality of sexual dimorphism and how we can we best deal with such aspects of our evolved biology in the contemporary world (Bachiochi 2021; Perry 2022; Harrington 2023).

The Jungians discussed in this chapter such as Ulanov, Neumann and Perera, who adopt Jung's concept of sexual difference, are more in accord with Finnegan's ethnographically informed analysis than those Jungians inspired by poststructuralist and postmodern feminist approaches. The latter – for example, the works of Samuels, Rowland, Gardner and Gray – represent a peculiarly Western intellectual and ideological orientation that has very little utility in explaining the ethnographic data nor the reality of evolved sex-based differences. I now turn to the scientific evidence for those differences.

The Ontogeny and Phylogeny of Sex Differences

It is clear from Jung's writings that he would have been opposed to social constructionism, deconstruction and the associated rejection of Eros and Logos as expressions of oppressive Enlightenment binary thinking. The fundamental premise of his psychology is that humans are not born as a *tabula rasa* or blank slate upon which culture inscribes its meanings (Stevens 2004: 248–50). His entire oeuvre is premised on the notion of archaic, subcortical brain systems that evolved before we became human, but which nevertheless inform our contemporary psychology.

For example, when children are born they already have biologically evolved predispositions that channel and constrain subsequent development. Jung was fully aware of this when he writes that the 'psyche of the child in its preconscious state is anything but a *tabula rasa*; it is already preformed in a recognizably individual way, and is moreover equipped with all specifically human instincts, as well as with the a priori foundations of the higher functions' (Jung 2011: 348). For Jung, this phylogenetic inheritance is established in utero; as he writes the '… brain is produced in each embryo in all its differentiated perfection, and when it starts functioning it will unfailingly produce the same results that have been produced innumerable times before in the ancestral line' (Jung 2014b: 480). Sex differences are part of this ancient evolutionary inheritance with the anima and animus representing the 'foundation stones of the psychic structure, which in its totality exceeds the limits of consciousness' (Jung et al. 1953: 20).

Modern research confirms these observations of Jung's. One of the many ways researchers seek to control for the relative influence of cultural variables and biological predispositions is by seeking to measure sex differences in infants prior to socialisation. For example, if sex differences are a result of socialisation, then they would not yet exist in neonates. In order to address this issue, researchers tested for sex differences in neonatal social perception (Connellan et al. 2000). The infants were only one day old; yet still at this early stage of development, male infants show a stronger interest in physical-mechanical objects while the female infants showed a stronger interest in faces. The authors conclude that their study clearly demonstrates 'that sex differences are in part biological in origin' (Connellan et al. 2000: 113). This is exactly what we would predict if the embryo is formed in utero and develops according to phylogenetic inheritance – that it brings with it inherited predispositions from the ancestral line as Jung argued. If the brain were a *tabula rasa* these differences would not be observed at such an early age before culture had a chance to mould psychological dispositions.

The greater preference female neonates tend to have for faces, and of males for mechanical or physical objects, is most likely related to sex-based differences in interests that also manifest in later periods of development. Similar differences have been found in older infants with males more likely than females to imitate propulsive movements, suggesting male sex-typed behaviour may develop from socialisation mechanisms that build on an evolved male predisposition to imitate propulsive motion (Benenson, Tennyson, and Wrangham 2011). The early emerging preference for faces in female newborns may be related to greater female proficiency in theory of mind and the ability to read emotional states from nonverbal cues such as facial expression (Carter, Hall, and Horgan 2000; McClure 2000; Benenson, Webb, and Wrangham 2022). This is most likely related to what researchers term the empathy quotient which females score higher on than males (Baron-Cohen and Wheelwright 2004)

These differences are most likely related to the 'animate' versus 'things' dichotomy in which females on average have higher levels of empathy and interest in relating to animate phenomena (people and animals) while males on average prefer mechanical objects and abstract systematising with greater ability for complex pattern recognition (Connellan et al. 2000; Baron-Cohen 2003, 2020; Ruigrok et al. 2014). In a study of half a million people, typical females on average showed higher levels of empathy with typical males on average showing higher levels of autistic and systematising traits. Females were also much more likely to be extreme empathisers, males more likely to be extreme systematisers while autistic people of both sexes showed a more masculinised profile (Greenberg et al. 2018). The systematising ability of the more masculinised brain is believed to underpin human inventiveness, creativity as well as the unusual abilities of the highly systemising autistic mind – abilities which may have been under selection for tens if not hundreds of thousands of years as more complex tools and weaponry were being invented which require systematising forms of cognition to manufacture. In this sense the systematising mind may have been crucial to our evolutionary success as a species (Baron-Cohen 2020). As noted above, Neumann associated Logos with patriarchal consciousness and enhanced systematising abilities, arguing that 'archetypally masculine consciousness is a most significant and, as the development of *Homo sapiens* shows, exceedingly successful organ of adaptation and information processing' (Neumann 1994: 93).

Some researchers have argued these differences manifest themselves in sex-based differences in occupational interests and achievement, cognitive and academic abilities as well as motivation for different areas of study and employment (Geary 2010; Su, Murdock and Rounds 2015; Stoet and Geary 2018). Importantly, females seem to have a bias towards the humanities and the life sciences (psychology and biology) which at the population level they prefer more than science, mathematics and technology. This suggests that it may not be lack of ability that results in these differences, but differences in interests and motivational proclivities, which are likely linked to biologically evolved sex differences in psychology (Stewart-Williams and Halsey 2021).

Interestingly, much of the research in this book derives from the pioneering primate field studies undertaken by women. Research pioneers like Jane Goodall and Diane Fossey paved the way for female scientists who now are major contributors to the fields of comparative primatology and human evolutionary studies. In fact, I would argue the most interesting research in the last few decades has been undertaken by women. This is not to say that women cannot excel in mathematics and physics – they obviously do. But not at the rate that males do. Significantly, in fields like psychology which focus on the interpersonal, female students graduate at approximately three times the rate of males (Gruber et al. 2021). More generally, in the life sciences such as biology and psychology, females seem to outperform males in terms of achievement and representation, which may be related to evolved differences in preferences and psychological orientation (Stewart-Williams and Halsey 2021).

Of course, as demonstrated in the gender similarity hypothesis, these are averages which means there is a great deal of overlap, with many males showing high degrees of empathy and many females being adept at, and interested in, abstract reasoning (Hyde 2005). The important point however, is the population level averages, and why more males prefer abstract systematising and occupy the extremes of the distribution, whereas females show a very strong population level bias towards empathic engagement with people and living things. It is worth noting that it is not only averages that are important, for example males show greater variation, which means they occupy the extremes of the distribution. This means that there are many more men who have lower intelligence than women – but also a large number who score higher than women. In other words, women tend to cluster more around the mean, whereas males have much greater variance which may be related to different evolutionary pressures on women versus men (Arden and Plomin 2006).

In mate preferences, the psychology of males and females also shows significant differences, which is most likely related to different reproductive strategies – for example, the costs of pregnancy are much higher for women than men as women are the sex who gestate the foetus and give birth. This would imply that females may be more circumspect when engaging in sex and prefer different qualities in a mate than males do as the consequences of intercourse are vastly different for each sex (Buss 2010; Walter et al. 2020).

While the above differences are significant, the most pronounced aspects of human sexual dimorphism are evident in motor behaviours such as throwing (Hyde 2005). Associated with throwing is male physical strength and particularly upper body strength and hand grip strength which is much greater than women's. While these differences are not particularly pronounced in children, when males enter puberty, their upper body and hand grip strength increases relative to that of females.

For example, large increases in lean body mass emerge with the development of secondary sexual characteristic in males but not females (Kirchengast 2010) with upper body muscle mass being approximately seventy five times higher in men than women (Lassek and Gaulin 2009). Additionally, biology plays a role in sex differences in throwing (Thomas and French 1985) with male upper body strength being up to twice that of female athletes (Bartolomei et al. 2021). As Joyce Benenson summarises these differences and their cross-cultural prevalence:

> Puberty causes boys to grow so much heavier, taller, and more muscular than girls that there is almost no overlap between the two sexes in these physical skills. Before adolescence, boys differ little from girls in their height, weight, muscle mass, and physical skills, except of course for throwing. The difference in throwing force and velocity occurs even in the tiniest hunter-gatherer communities.
> (Benenson 2014: 28)

It is uncertain why these differences exist. One factor may be that females most likely did not need to engage in physical conflict as much as males in our evolutionary past. In primate species males will often attack predators such as leopards while females and their infants seek protection in trees (Kummer et al. 1967: 154–5; Lin et al. 2020: 11).The fact that over evolutionary time, females are the sex that nurtured and fed vulnerable infants, may have made them more temperamentally averse to the presence of violence and conflict, as such conflict would endanger both themselves and the lives of their vulnerable offspring. Conversely, it is possible that hominin males required greater physical strength to protect the group from external threat. With the advent of tools and weaponry such as spears selection for greater upper body strength and hand grip would have also been favoured in males – for hunting, predator defence and possibly in interpersonal conflict (Young 2003; Isen, McGue and Iacono 2014).

While some primates can throw projectiles humans are unique in the degree of accuracy they are able to do so. Throwing projectiles in the manner humans do seems to result from several unique anatomical features enabling elastic energy storage and release at the shoulder. Fossil evidence suggests these features first appeared together approximately 2 million years ago in the species *Homo erectus* when we begin to see increased archaeological evidence for both tool manufacture and hunting and that consequently selection for throwing as a means to hunt probably had an important role in the evolution of the genus *Homo* (Roach et al. 2013).

Benenson has argued that this evolutionary trend is also associated with the male role as group protectors against abstract enemies, the enemy that 'wakes people in the night' and that seeks 'to destroy you and all that you love' (Benenson 2014: 29). The fantasies of young boys, as well as their preferred play activities– which differ markedly from girls – involve cooperation between groups of male friends who collectively seek to protect the group from harm. Benenson suggests this is the basis of unique forms of male sociality, cooperation and group level cognition and affect which differs from that which is found in girls and women (Benenson 2014: 30–42). Additionally, Benenson argues that women often support men in this behaviour and expect men to collectively fight enemies that threaten the safety of the group (Benenson 2014: 25). In our ancestral past, such group defence, against either predators who are known to have influenced hominin evolution (Treves and Palmqvist 2007) or other hostile humans, would have been crucial for survival. It is no wonder that young boy's and men's minds are attuned to protecting the group in such a manner. Not having to nurse and feed infants they were the sex that evolved extra body strength and muscle mass in order to protect infants, children and their mothers. Such sex differences, when combined in a cohesive social group, make for a dynamic and complimentary partnership. This is most likely the deep evolutionary of origin of Eros and Logos.

Young girls and women tend to develop different kinds of relationships than young boys and men, focussing on support networks and alliances that can assist them in child rearing and resist the potential threats posed by males who are neither kin nor allies (Power, Sommer, and Watts 2013; Benenson et al. 2022). It is these sex-specific psychologies that most likely underpin differences in the development of boys and girls noted above by Ulanov and Neumann. Anthropologist Carolyn Edwards has argued that the different play preferences of boys versus girls, as well

as different forms of social orientation, are not necessarily due to external socialisation, but self-socialisation driven by biological predispositions. As she writes:

> The system of self-socialisation is founded on attraction to like-sex community
> members followed by identification. Girls are predisposed in their development
> to maintain proximity to adult females, where they receive maximal opportunity
> to attend selectively and maintain proximity to infants, with the result that they
> gain knowledge and practice in nurturing styles of interaction. As they gain
> knowledge and practice, they become more skilled caregivers, with the result
> that nurturant interaction becomes differentially rewarding to them.
>
> (Edwards 2002: 337)

One of the assertions of social constructionists is that these differences are the
result of cultural influences. This is to a degree a valid point as culture and socialisation do play an important role. To control for cultural variables researchers have
looked to a broad range of societies, from hunter-gatherers to pastoralists and modern industrial societies. This research focusses on childhood sex-segregated play
groups, toy preferences and their relationship to adult social roles. Researchers
have also investigated sex differences in primates. If we find differences that exist
cross-culturally, and also in our primate cousins, then this suggests they are part of
our deep phylogenetic inheritance as Jung argued. It is through these cross-cultural
and cross-species forms of analysis that researchers have sought to test the validity
of the social constructionist hypotheses.

For example, one of the claims made by social constructionists is that gender-
typical toy preferences are products of socialisation and parental influence (Boe
and Woods 2018). This is unlikely to be the full explanation. Evidence suggests
that sex-based play behaviours are part of our primate and mammalian heritage.
For example, ludic impulses are common among mammals and may function to
facilitate the expression of joy, cooperation and the limits and nature of social hierarchies – they are also more likely to occur when juveniles are in a safe and pro-
tective environment free of fear and hunger (Panksepp 2004: 280–1). While play
behaviour in young children seems to show a gender difference cross-culturally
and the nature of those differences varies, some form of sex-based difference seems
to be universal. In other words, there seems to be no human culture in which male
and female toy and play preferences are identical. This suggests that evolutionary
factors may be interacting with the social and physical environment (Fry 2005).

One of the most pronounced gender differences in play is boys have a greater
preference for vigorous forms of rough and tumble play or play fighting (DiPietro
1981). While this trend exists cross-culturally, it is likely that such evolved sex-
based predispositions interact with environmental factors giving rise to 'variations
on a the theme' (Fry 2005: 55). One variation upon this theme is found among the
Hadza, a hunter-gatherer people of Tanzania in Africa. Hadza boys are given bows
and arrows from as early as two to three years of age with every male being given
them by six years of age (Marlowe 2010: 84). Another is found among Indigenous

communities in Brazil where young boys engage in mock fighting against one another as well as small animals (Gosso et al. 2005).

Commenting on sexually dimorphic toy preferences in humans, it has been argued that 'sexually differentiated object preferences' may have arisen early in human evolution 'prior to the emergence of a distinct [hominin] lineage.' This suggests that such sex-based preferences may be part of the deep 'primate layer' in the human psyche Jung believed we inherit from our evolutionary past (Jung 2020: 202). As the authors continue such preferences may have evolved from 'differential selection pressures based on the different behavioural roles of males and females, and that evolved object feature preferences may contribute to present day sexually dimorphic toy preferences in children' (Alexander and Hines 2002).

Other evidence for the phylogenesis of sex differences in toy preferences comes from studies of juvenile primates. Intriguingly, young female chimpanzees have been observed engaging in a form of play-mothering, carrying sticks in a manner suggestive of rudimentary doll play (Kahlenberg and Wrangham 2010). Significantly, this behaviour occurs prior to the first birth, involves carrying the sticks into the night nest and was not observed once a female had given birth. Such play behaviour seems to be consistent with practice for adult roles. Based on these findings, it has been argued that a similar 'sex difference could have occurred in the human and pre-human lineage at least since our common ancestry with chimpanzees, well before direct socialisation became an important influence (Kahlenberg and Wrangham 2010: 1068).

At the start of this chapter, I quoted Jung's assertion that his theory of sexual polarity is based on 'masculine and feminine genes' (Jung 2014a: 175). In evolutionary terms, genetic differences in the present are often a result of a long evolutionary history with extensive phylogenetic depth reaching into the ancient past – what I called in Chapter 1 'deep time.' In the above discussion I explored a few examples from the vast literature on evolved sex-based differences. There is also a significant body of modern research that supports Jung's contention of genetically based differences between males and females, not just in anatomy but also in psychology and social and sexual behaviour. This literature is a valuable resource for Jungian scholars seeking to extend Jung's evolutionary conception of evolved sex differences (for extensive reviews, see Geary 2010; Pinker 2010; Benenson 2014; Konner 2015; Buss 2021; de Waal 2022).

Some important recent research into the genetics of sex-based differences include the identification of genes that show sex biased expression throughout development, from the prenatal period to adulthood (Shi, Zhang, and Su 2016). There also appears to be genes involved in sex-biased brain anatomy and development that humans share with other mammals, suggesting that sex differences are very ancient in evolutionary terms and conserved among a wide range of animal species (Liu et al. 2020). Significantly, while there are thousands of genes that have sex biased expression at all developmental stages the largest number appear to be expressed during puberty. Importantly, there appears to be enrichment of male biased genes associated with neurological and psychiatric disorders like schizophrenia, bipolar disorder, Alzheimer's disease and autism, while such a pattern does not seem to appear for the female-biased genes (Shi et al. 2016). This research provides confirmatory evidence for Jung's view on the influence of genetic factors on sex-based psychological differences quoted at the start of this chapter (Jung 2014a: 175).

Primatologist Franz De Waal has discussed much of this evidence at length in his book *Different: What Apes Can Teach us About Gender*. It is a book that Jungians interested in evolutionary approaches to analytical psychology would benefit immensely from reading. De Waal discusses social constructionism and Judith Butler's assertion that because 'gender is not a fact, the various acts of gender create the idea of gender, and without those acts, there would be no gender at all' (Butler 1988: 522). De Waal rejects this assertion and provides his own definition of gender, which he contrasts with Butler's: 'Gender refers to the learned overlays that turn a biological female into a woman and a biological male into a man' (de Waal 2022: 12).

De Waal elaborates on this idea, writing that sex differences that emerge in early life such as the 'high level of energy and roughhousing of young males' and the attraction 'to dolls, infants and babysitting of young females' are variations on similar behaviours evident in 'most mammals, from rats to dogs and from elephants to whales.' It evolved, he continues, thanks to the 'distinct ways the sexes transmit their genes to the next generation' (de Waal 2022: 311). And when discussing the notion that the passion that young girls have for infants and dolls is stereotypical, he writes:

> Its time … to stop calling the passion of girls for infants and dolls stereotypical. Human behaviour that is found all over the world and shared with many other mammals isn't explained by prejudice and gender expectations, even though they may contribute. It goes deeper than that. Biology is involved, and for a good reason. Since maternal skills are too complex to be left to instinct, evolution made sure that the gender that needs them most is eager to get maternity training …. A tendency that is functionally tied to an age-old mode of reproduction isn't stereotypical but *archetypical*.
>
> (de Waal 2022: 268; italics in original)

References

Alexander, G., and M. Hines. 2002. 'Sex Differences in Response to Children's Toys in Nonhuman Primates (Cercopithecus aethiops sabaeus)', *Evolution and Human Behavior*, 23: 467–79.

Arden, R., and R. Plomin. 2006. 'Sex Differences in Variance of Intelligence across Childhood', *Personality and Individual Differences*, 41: 39–48.

Bachiochi, E. 2021. *The Rights of Women: Reclaiming a Lost Vision* (University of Notre Dame Press).

Baron-Cohen, S. 2003. *Men, Women and the Extreme Male Brain* (University of Michigan).

Baron-Cohen, S. 2020. *The Pattern Seekers: A New Theory of Human Invention* (Penguin Books Limited).

Baron-Cohen, S., and S. Wheelwright. 2004. 'The Empathy Quotient: An Investigation of Adults with Asperger Syndrome or High Functioning Autism, and Normal Sex Differences', *Journal of Autism and Developmental Disorders*, 34: 163–75.

Bartels, A., and S. Zeki. 2004. 'The Neural Correlates of Maternal and Romantic Love', *NeuroImage*, 21: 1155–66.

Bartolomei, S., G. Grillone, R. Di Michele, and M. Cortesi. 2021. 'A Comparison between Male and Female Athletes in Relative Strength and Power Performances', *Journal of Functional Morphology and Kinesiology*, 6: 1–11.

Benenson, J. 2014. *Warriors and Worriers: The Survival of the Sexes* (OUP USA).

Benenson, J. 2019. 'Sex Differences in Primate Social Relationships during Development.' in Welling, L.L.M., and T.K. Shackelford (eds.), *The Oxford Handbook of Evolutionary Psychology and Behavioral Endocrinology* (Oxford University Press).

Benenson, J., R. Tennyson, and R. Wrangham. 2011. 'Male More than Female Infants Imitate Propulsive Motion', *Cognition*, 121: 262–7.

Benenson, J., C. Webb, and R. Wrangham. 2022. 'Self-Protection as an Adaptive Female Strategy', *Behavioral and Brain Sciences*, 45: e128.

Bishop, P. 2007. *Analytical Psychology and German Classical Aesthetics: Goethe, Schiller, and Jung, Volume 1: The Development of the Personality* (Taylor & Francis).

Bishop, P. 2008. *Analytical Psychology and German Classical Aesthetics: Goethe, Schiller, and Jung Volume 2: The Constellation of the Self* (Taylor & Francis).

Boe, J.L., and R.J. Woods. 2018. 'Parents' Influence on Infants' Gender-Typed Toy Preferences', *Sex Roles*, 79: 358–73.

Buss, D. 2010. 'Sex Differences in Human Mate Preferences: Evolutionary Hypotheses Tested in 37 Cultures', *Behavioral and Brain Sciences*, 12: 1–14.

Buss, D.M. 2021. *Bad Men: The Hidden Roots of Sexual Deception, Harassment and Assault* (Little, Brown Book Group).

Butler, J. 1988. 'Performative Acts and Gender Constitution: An Essay in Phenomenology and Feminist Theory', *Theatre Journal*, 40: 519–31.

Butler, J. 2011. *Gender Trouble: Feminism and the Subversion of Identity* (Taylor & Francis).

Carhart-Harris, R.L., R. Leech, P.J. Hellyer, M. Shanahan, A. Feilding, E. Tagliazucchi, et al. 2014. 'The Entropic Brain: A Theory of Conscious States Informed by Neuroimaging Research with Psychedelic Drugs', *Frontiers in Human Neuroscience*, 8: 1–22.

Carter, J., J. Hall, and T. Horgan. 2000. 'Gender Differences in Nonverbal Communication of Emotion.' in Fischer, A.H. (ed.), *Gender and Emotion: Social Psychological Perspectives* (Cambridge University Press).

Casiraghi, L., I. Spiousas, G. Dunster, K. McGlothlen, E. Fernández-Duque, C Valeggia, et al. 2021. 'Moonstruck Sleep: Synchronization of Human Sleep with the Moon Cycle under Field Conditions', *Science Advances*, 7: eabe0465.

Cepeda, I., M. Lacalle-Calderon, and M. Torralba. 2022. 'Measuring Violence against Women: A Global Index', *Journal of Interpersonal Violence*, 37: NP18614-NP38.

Chiari, S. 2018. *Shakespeare's Representation of Weather, Climate and Environment: The Early Modern 'Fated Sky'* (Edinburgh University Press).

Clark, G. 2020. 'Carl Jung, John Layard and Jordan Peterson: Assessing Theories of Human Social Evolution and Their Implications for Analytical Psychology', *International Journal of Jungian Studies*, 12: 129–58.

Clark, G. 2021. 'Carl Jung and the Psychedelic Brain: An Evolutionary Model of Analytical Psychology Informed by Psychedelic Neuroscience', *International Journal of Jungian Studies*, 14(2): 1–30.

Clark, G. 2022. 'The Dionysian Primate: Goethe, Nietzsche, Jung and Psychedelic Neuroscience.' in Miils, J., and D. Burston (eds.), *Psychoanalysis and the Mind-Body Problem* (Routledge).

Connellan, J., S. Baron-Cohen, S. Wheelwright, A. Batki, and J. Ahluwalia. 2000. 'Sex Differences in Human Neonatal Social Perception', *Infant Behavior and Development*, 23: 113–8.

Daly, M., and M. Wilson. 1990. 'Killing the Competition: Female/Female and Male/Male Homicide', *Human Nature*, 1: 81–107.

de Waal, F. 2022. *Different: What Apes Can Teach Us about Gender* (Granta Publications).

Derrida, J. 2016. *Of Grammatology* (Johns Hopkins University Press).

Diogo, R. 2024. *Darwin's Racism, Sexism, and Idolization: Their Tragic Societal and Scientific Repercussions* (Springer Nature Switzerland).

DiPietro, J. 1981. 'Rough and Tumble Play: A Function of Gender', *Developmental Psychology*, 17: 50.

Dissanayake, E. 2021. 'Ancestral Human Mother-Infant Interaction Was an Adaptation that Gave Rise to Music and Dance', *Behavioral and Brain Sciences*, 44: e68.

Douglas, C. 2000. *The Woman in the Mirror: Analytical Psychology and the Feminine* (iUniverse).

Edinger, E.F. 1990. *Goethe's Faust: Notes for a Jungian Commentary* (Inner City Books).

Edwards, C.P. 2002. 'Behavioral Sex Differences in Children of Diverse Cultures.' in Pereira, M.E. (ed.), *Juvenile Primates: Life History, Development and Behavior* (University of Chicago Press).

Finnegan, M. 2013. 'The Politics of Eros: Ritual Dialogue and Egalitarianism in Three Central African Hunter-Gatherer Societies', *Journal of the Royal Anthropological Institute*, 19: 697–715.

Freud, S., J. Strachey, and A. Freud. 2001. *The Complete Psychological Works of Sigmund Freud Vol.18: Beyond the Pleasure Principle-Group Psychology & Other Works* (Random House UK).

Fry, D.P. 2005. 'Rough-and-Tumble Social Play in Humans.' in Pellegrini, D., and P.K. Smith (eds.), *The Nature of Play: Great Apes and Humans* (Guilford Press).

Gardner, L., and F. Gray. 2016. *Feminist Views from Somewhere: Post-Jungian Themes in Feminist Theory* (Taylor & Francis).

Geary, D.C. 2010. *Male, Female: The Evolution of Human Sex Differences* (American Psychological Association).

Gimbutas, M. 2001. *The Language of the Goddess: Unearthing the Hidden Symbols of Western Civilization* (Thames & Hudson).

Glasper, E.R., W.M. Kenkel, J. Bick, and J.K. Rilling. 2019. 'More than Just Mothers: The Neurobiological and Neuroendocrine Underpinnings of Allomaternal Caregiving', *Frontiers in Neuroendocrinology*, 53: 100741.

Goodall, J. 1986. *The Chimpanzees of Gombe: Patterns of Behavior* (Belknap Press of Harvard University Press).

Goodall, J. 1996. *In the Shadow of Man* (Phoenix).

Gosso, Y., E. Otta, M. de Lima Salum e Morais, F.J.L. Ribeiro, and V.S.R. Bussab. 2005. 'Play in Hunter-Gatherer Society.' in Pellegrini, D., and P.K. Smith (eds.), *The Nature of Play: Great Apes and Humans* (Guilford Press).

Gould, S.J., and E.S. Vrba. 1982. 'Exaptation-A Missing Term in the Science of Form', *Paleobiology*, 8: 4–15.

Gowaty, P.A. 1992. 'Evolutionary Biology and Feminism', *Human Nature*, 3: 217–49.

Gowaty, P.A. 2003. 'Power Asymmetries between the Sexes, Mate Preferences, and Components of Fitness.' in Brown, T.C. (ed.), *Evolution, Gender, and Rape* (MIT Press).

Gowaty, P.A. 2012. *Feminism and Evolutionary Biology: Boundaries, Intersections and Frontiers* (Springer Science & Business Media).

Greenberg, D.M., V. Warrier, C. Allison, and S. Baron-Cohen. 2018. 'Testing the Empathizing-Systemizing Theory of Sex Differences and the Extreme Male Brain Theory of Autism in Half a Million People', *Proceedings of the National Academy of Sciences of the United States of America*, 115: 12152–7.

Gruber, J., J. Mendle, K.A. Lindquist, T. Schmader, L.A. Clark, and E. Bliss-Moreau, et al. 2021. 'The Future of Women in Psychological Science', *Perspectives on Psychological Science*, 16: 483–516.

Hager, L. 2005. *Women in Human Evolution* (Taylor & Francis).

Harding, M.E. 1936. *Woman's Mysteries: Ancient and Modern* (Longman).

Harrington, M. 2023. *Feminism against Progress* (Forum).

Hauke, C. 2000. *Jung and the Postmodern: The Interpretation of Realities* (Routledge).

Hawkes, K., and J.E. Coxworth 2013. 'Grandmothers and the Evolution of Human Longevity: A Review of Findings and Future Directions', *Evolutionary Anthropology*, 22: 294–302.

Helfrich-Förster, C., S. Monecke, I. Spiousas, T. Hovestadt, O. Mitesser, and T.A. Wehr. 2021. 'Women Temporarily Synchronize Their Menstrual Cycles with the Luminance and Gravimetric Cycles of the Moon', *Science Advances*, 7: eabe1358.

Hobson, A. 1999. *Dreaming as Delirium: How the Brain Goes Out of Its Mind* (MIT Press).

Hobson, A. 2014. *Psychodynamic Neurology: Dreams, Consciousness, and Virtual Reality* (Taylor & Francis).

Hobson, A., C.C.H. Hong, and K.J. Friston. 2014. 'Virtual Reality and Consciousness Inference in Dreaming', *Frontiers in Psychology*, 5: 1–18.

Hrdy, S.B. 1999. *The Woman That Never Evolved: With a New Preface and Bibliographical Updates, Revised Edition* (Harvard University Press).

Hrdy, S.B. 2000. *Mother Nature: Maternal Instincts and How They Shape the Human Species* (Ballantine Books).

Hrdy, S.B. 2009. *Mothers and Others: The Evolutionary Origins of Mutual Understanding* (Belknap Press of Harvard University Press).

Hyde, J. S. 2005. 'The Gender Similarities Hypothesis', *American Psychologist*, 60: 581–92.

Isen, J., M. McGue, and W. Iacono. 2014. 'Genetic Influences on the Development of Grip Strength in Adolescence', *American Journal of Physical Anthropology*, 154: 189–200.

Jung, C.G. 1953. *Collected Works of C.G. Jung, Volume 9 (Part 2): Aion Researches Into the Phenomenology of the Self* (Princeton University Press).

Jung, C.G. 1960. *The Collected Works of C.G. Jung: The Psychogenesis of Mental Disease* (Routledge & Kegan Paul).

Jung, C.G. 1983. *The Psychology of the Transference* (Routledge).

Jung, C.G. 2011. *Memories, Dreams, Reflections* (Knopf Doubleday Publishing Group).

Jung, C.G. 2014a. *Collected Works of C.G. Jung, Volume 9 (Part 1): Archetypes and the Collective Unconscious* (Princeton University Press).

Jung, C.G. 2014b. *The Structure and Dynamics of the Psyche* (Taylor & Francis).

Jung, C.G. 2014c. *Symbols of Transformation* (Taylor & Francis).

Jung, C.G. 2020. *C.G. Jung Speaking: Interviews and Encounters* (Princeton University Press).

Jung, C.G., and G. Adler. 2014. *The Development of Personality* (Taylor & Francis).

Jung, C.G., H. Read, R.F.C. Hull, M. Fordham, and G. Adler. 1953. *Collected Works of C.G. Jung, Volume 9 (Part 2): Aion Researches Into the Phenomenology of the Self* (Princeton University Press).

Kahlenberg, S.M., and R.W. Wrangham. 2010. 'Sex Differences in chimpanzees' Use of Sticks as Play Objects Resemble Those of Children', *Current Biology*, 20: R1067–R68.

Kirchengast, S. 2010. 'Gender Differences in Body Composition from Childhood to Old Age: An Evolutionary Point of View', *Journal of Life Sciences*, 2: 1–10.

Knight, C. 1995. *Blood Relations: Menstruation and the Origins of Culture* (Yale University Press).

Knight, C., and J. Lewis. 2016. 'Towards a Theory of Everything.' in Power, C., M. Finnegan, and H. Calla (eds.), *Human Origins: Contributions from Social Anthropology* (Berghahn Books).

Knight, C. 1988. 'Menstrual Synchrony and the Australian Rainbow Snake.' in Buckley, T., and A. Gottlieb (eds.), *Blood Magic: The Anthropology of Menstruation* (University of California Press).

Konner, M. 2015. *Women after All: Sex, Evolution, and the End of Male Supremacy* (W. W. Norton).

Kramer, K.L. 2005. 'Children's Help and the Pace of Reproduction: Cooperative Breeding in Humans', *Evolutionary Anthropology: Issues*, 14: 224–37.

Kronfeld-Schor, N., D. Dominoni, H. de la Iglesia, O. Levy, E.D. Herzog, T. Dayan, et al. 2013. 'Chronobiology by Moonlight', *Proceedings of the Royal Society B: Biological Sciences*, 280: 20123088.

Kummer, H., H.O. Hofer, A.H. Schultz, and D. Starck. 1967. *Social Organization of Hamadryas Baboons: A Field Study* (S. Karger AG).

Lassek, William D., and Steven J.C. Gaulin. 2009. 'Costs and Benefits of Fat-Free Muscle Mass in Men: Relationship to Mating Success, Dietary Requirements, and Native Immunity', *Evolution and Human Behavior*, 30: 322–28.

Lawick-Goodall, Jane van. 1968. 'The Behaviour of Free-Living Chimpanzees in the Gombe Stream Reserve', *Animal Behaviour Monographs*, 1: 161–311.

Lee, R.B. 1979. *The! Kung San: Men, Women and Work in a Foraging Society* (Cambridge University Press).

Lewis, J. 2008. 'Ekila: Blood, Bodies, and Egalitarian Societies', *Journal of the Royal Anthropological Institute*, 14: 297–315.

Lin, B., I.R. Foxfoot, C.M. Miller, V.V. Venkatamaran, J.T. Kerby, E.K. Bechtold, et al. 2020. 'Leopard Predation on Gelada Monkeys at Guassa, Ethiopia', *American Journal of Primatology*, 82: e23098.

Liu, S., J. Seidlitz, J.D. Blumenthal, L.S. Clasen, and A. Raznahan. 2020. 'Integrative Structural, Functional, and Transcriptomic Analyses of Sex-Biased Brain Organization in Humans', *Proceedings of the National Academy of Sciences of the United States of America*, 117: 18788–98.

Maestripieri, D., and S. Pelka. 2002. 'Sex Differences in Interest in Infants across the Lifespan', *Human Nature*, 13: 327–44.

Marlowe, F. 2010. *The Hadza: Hunter-Gatherers of Tanzania* (University of California Press).

McClure, E.B. 2000. 'A Meta-Analytic Review of Sex Differences in Facial Expression Processing and Their Development in Infants, Children, and Adolescents', *Psychological Bulletin*, 126: 424.

Munn, N.D. 1984. 'The Transformation of Subjects into Objects in Walbiri and Pitjantjatjara Myth.' in Charlesworth, M.J. (ed.), *Religion in Aboriginal Australia: An Anthology* (University of Queensland Press).

Murphy, M.R., J.R. Seckl, S. Burton, S.A. Checkley, and S.L. Lightman. 1987. 'Changes in Oxytocin and Vasopressin Secretion during Sexual Activity in Men', *The Journal of Clinical Endocrinology & Metabolism*, 65: 738–41.

Nagy, M. 1981. 'Menstruation and Shamanism', *Psychological Perspectives*, 12: 52–68.

Neumann, E. 1994. *The Fear of the Feminine: And Other Essays on Feminine Psychology* (Princeton University Press).

Nichols, D.E. 2013. 'Serotonin, and the Past and Future of LSD', *MAPS Bulletin Special Edition*.

O'Connell, J.F., K. Hawkes, and N.G. Blurton Jones. 1999. 'Grandmothering and the Evolution of Homo erectus', *Journal of Human Evolution*, 36: 461–85.

Panksepp, J., and L. Biven. 2012. *The Archaeology of Mind: Neuroevolutionary Origins of Human Emotions* (W. W. Norton).

Panksepp, J. 2004. *Affective Neuroscience: The Foundations of Human and Animal Emotions* (Oxford University Press).

Perera, S.B. 1981. *Descent to the Goddess: A Way of Initiation for Women* (Inner City Books).

Perry, L. 2022. *The Case against the Sexual Revolution* (Polity Press).

Phoenix, J. 2023. 'Sex, Gender, Identity and Criminology.' in Todd, S., and A. Sullivan (eds.), *Sex and Gender: A Contemporary Reader* (Routledge).

Pinker, S. 2010. *The Sexual Paradox: Extreme Men, Gifted Women and the Real Gender Gap* (Random House of Canada).

Power, C. 2022a. 'Lunarchy: The Original Human Economics of Time.' in Silva, F., and L. Henty (eds.), *Solarizing the Moon: Essays in Honour of Lionel Sims* (Archaeopress).

Power, C., V. Sommer, and I. Watts. 2013. 'The Seasonality Thermostat: Female Reproductive Synchrony and Male Behavior in Monkeys, Neanderthals, and Modern Humans', *PaleoAnthropology*, 2013: 33–60.

Power, C. 2017. 'Reconstructing a Source Cosmology for African Hunter-Gatherers.' in Power, C., M. Finnegan, and H. Calla (eds.), *Human Origins: Contributions from Social Anthropology* (Berghahn Books).

Roach, N.T., M. Venkadesan, M.J. Rainbow, and D.E. Lieberman. 2013. 'Elastic Energy Storage in the Shoulder and the Evolution of High-Speed Throwing in Homo', *Nature*, 498: 483–6.

Rowland, S. 2004. 'Jung's Ghost Stories: Jung for Literary Theory in Feminism, Poststructuralism, and Postmodernism.' in Baumlin, J., T. Baumlin, and G. Jensen (eds.), *Post-Jungian Criticism: Theory and Practice* (State University of New York Press).

Rowland, S. 2002. *Jung: A Feminist Revision* (Wiley).

Ruigrok, A.N., G. Salimi-Khorshidi, M.C. Lai, S. Baron-Cohen, M.V. Lombardo, R.J. Tait, et al. 2014. 'A Meta-Analysis of Sex Differences in Human Brain Structure', *Neuroscience & Biobehavioral Reviews*, 39: 34–50.

Samuels, A. 2016. *The Plural Psyche: Personality, Morality and the Father* (Taylor & Francis).

Seung, T.K. 2006. *Goethe, Nietzsche, and Wagner: Their Spinozan Epics of Love and Power* (Lexington Books).

Shi, L., Z. Zhang, and B. Su. 2016. 'Sex Biased Gene Expression Profiling of Human Brains at Major Developmental Stages', *Scientific Reports*, 6: 21181.

Smuts, B.B. 2017. *Sex and Friendship in Baboons* (Taylor & Francis).

Sosis, R., H.C. Kress, and J.S. Boster. 2007. 'Scars for War: Evaluating Alternative Signaling Explanations for Cross-Cultural Variance in Ritual Costs', *Evolution and Human Behavior*, 28: 234–47.

Stevens, A. 2002. *Archetype Revisited: An Updated Natural History of the Self* (Brunner-Routledge).

Stevens, A. 2004. *Archetype Revisited: An Updated Natural History of the Self* (Taylor & Francis).

Stewart-Williams, S., and L.G. Halsey. 2021. 'Men, Women and STEM: Why the Differences and What Should Be Done?', *European Journal of Personality*, 35: 3–39.

Stock, K. 2023. 'Is Womanhood a Social Fact? in Todd, S., and A. Sullivan (eds.), *Sex and Gender: A Contemporary Reader* (Routledge).

Stoet, G., and D.C. Geary. 2018. 'The Gender-Equality Paradox in Science, Technology, Engineering, and Mathematics Education', *Psychological Science*, 29: 581–93.

Storey, A.E., C.J. Walsh, R.L. Quinton, and K.E. Wynne-Edwards. 2000. 'Hormonal Correlates of Paternal Responsiveness in New and Expectant Fathers', *Evolution and Human Behavior*, 21: 79–95.

Su, R., C. Murdock, and J. Rounds. 2015. 'Person-Environment Fit.' In Hartung, P.J., M. L. Savickas, and W.B. Walsh (eds.), *APA Handbook of Career Intervention, Volume 1: Foundations* (American Psychological Association).

Sullivan, A., and S. Todd. 2023. *Sex and Gender: A Contemporary Reader* (Taylor & Francis).

Tanner, N., and A. Zihlman. 1976. 'Women in Evolution. Part I: Innovation and Selection in Human Origins', *Signs*, 1: 585–608.

Thomas, J.R., and K.E. French. 1985. 'Gender Differences across Age in Motor Performance: A Meta-Analysis', *Psychological Bulletin*, 98: 260–82.

Treves, A., and P. Palmqvist. 2007. 'Reconstructing Hominin Interactions with Mammalian Carnivores (6.0–1.8 Ma).' in Gursky, S.L., and K.A.I. Nekaris (eds.), *Primate Anti-Predator Strategies* (Springer US).

Tucker, A. 2022. *Mom Genes: Inside the New Science of Our Ancient Maternal Instinct* (Gallery Books).

Ulanov, A.B. 1971. *The Feminine in Jungian Psychology and in Christian Theology* (Northwestern University Press).

Ulanov, A.B. 1981. *Receiving Woman: Studies in the Psychology and Theology of the Feminine* (Presbyterian Publishing Corporation).

VanderLaan, D.P., Z. Ren, and P.L. Vasey. 2013. 'Male Androphilia in the Ancestral Environment. An Ethnological Analysis', *Human Nature*, 24: 375–401.

Vasey, P.L., D.S. Pocock, and D.P. VanderLaan. 2007. 'Kin Selection and Male Androphilia in Samoan fa'afafine', *Evolution and Human Behavior*, 28: 159–67.

Walter, K.V., D. Conroy-Beam, D.M. Buss, K. Asao, and A. Sorokowska, P. Sorokowska, et al. 2020. 'Sex Differences in Mate Preferences across 45 Countries: A Large-Scale Replication', *Psychological Science*, 31: 408–23.

Wehr, D.S. 1987. *Jung and Feminism: Liberating Archetypes* (Beacon Press).

Whiting, B.B., C.P. Edwards, C.P. Edwards, and C.R. Ember. 1988. *Children of Different Worlds: The Formation of Social Behavior* (Harvard University Press).

Wollstonecraft, M., and M. Brody. 1992. *A Vindication of the Rights of Woman* (Penguin Books).

Wynne-Edwards, K.E. 2001. 'Hormonal Changes in Mammalian Fathers', *Hormones and Behavior*, 40: 139–45.

Wynne-Edwards, K.E., and C.J. Reburn. 2000. 'Behavioral Endocrinology of Mammalian Fatherhood', *Trends in Ecology & Evolution*, 15: 464–8.

Young, R.W. 2003. 'Evolution of the Human Hand: The Role of Throwing and Clubbing', *Journal of Anatomy*, 202: 165–74.

Chapter 4

Evolutionary Theory and Analytical Psychology

Introduction

In previous chapters, I have looked at various aspects of Jung's evolutionary thought, focussing on the historical contexts of its genesis, his engagement with anthropology and his views on evolved sex-based differences. In this chapter, I deepen that analysis by focussing on the fossil evidence for human evolution. This will take us back in time some 5 million years to Miocene Africa when the first evidence of hominin fossils appears.

The earliest hominins such as the small-brained *Ardipithecus ramidus* would have lacked a trajectory of brain development like modern humans, most likely reaching maturity much earlier than we do. It was not until later hominins such as *Homo erectus* that a human like ontogeny or life history pattern would have emerged, with an extended period of socio-cognitive development. This extended period of brain maturation is referred to as adolescence and during ontogeny this period involves the maturation of the default mode network, the emergence of adult like forms of ego consciousness and the transition from subcortical affect-based control of behaviour to more cortical forms of control. One of the probable consequences of the phylogenetic extension of human ontogeny and the evolution of an adolescent period of growth is that humans became much more susceptible to psychopathology than other primate species. Further, ritual life, and particularly adolescent initiation rites, may be cultural technologies designed to facilitate this difficult socio-cognitive transition.

I discuss the fossil evidence for the phylogenetic emergence of prosociality and a human pattern of brain development in the context of debates in theoretical biology. More specifically, I discuss debates regarding individual versus group-level selection as they pertain to the evolution of altruism and cooperation as well as the exaptation of the oxytocin system as a possible explanation for human prosociality.

Models of Human Sociality: Group Selection and Exaptation

In his *Darwin's Cathedral: Evolution, Religion, and the Nature of Society*, David Sloan Wilson develops a model of group selection to explain the highly cooperative nature of human sociality. Wilson argues that some of the major ideas in

DOI: 10.4324/9781032624549-5

Durkheim's *The Elementary Forms of Religious Life* find support from the findings of modern evolutionary theory. More specifically, he suggests that group-level adaptations, often facilitated by symbolic ritual activity, may have been adaptive throughout human evolution (Wilson 2003).

In *The Elementary Forms of Religious Life*, Durkheim connects kinship systems with ritual life and the way the formation of social groups is facilitated by symbolic representations. It is the connection between the sacred, symbolism and ritual life that Durkheim believes to be a fundamental feature of not only the elementary forms of religion such as totemism, but also religion more generally. As he writes:

> Religious representations are collective representations that express collective realities; rituals are ways of acting that are generated only within assembled groups and are meant to stimulate and sustain or recreate certain mental states in these groups. But if these categories of thought have religious origins, they must participate in what is common to all religious phenomena: they too must be social things, the products of collective thought.
>
> (Durkheim 2008: 11)

The issues raised by Sloan Wilson in his analysis of Durkheim are part of one of the major debates in theoretical biology. It concerns the evolution of altruism and cooperation which are crucial aspects of human social structure. Some of the questions involved are: how did social cooperation evolve through evolutionary processes if natural selection operates on the genes of individuals, can selection operate on social groups and are there more ancient neurobiological substrates involved in female mammalian nurturant behaviour that may form the basis of cooperation and altruism in humans?

One of the major theoretical innovations of modern biology is the concept of kin selection or inclusive fitness developed by evolutionary biologist William Hamilton (1936–2000). Hamilton was trying to understand altruism and cooperative behaviour which are seemingly anomalous phenomena if it is assumed that evolution is a process that favours the genes of individuals. Hamilton proposed that relatives share genes and that consequently there is a relationship between degree of relatedness and altruistic behaviour (Hamilton 1964a, 1964b).

The conceptual assumption behind inclusive fitness theory was summed up by a comment attributed to the biologist J.B.S. Haldane. One evening in a pub Haldane is said to have told his friends that he would 'jump into a river and risk his life to save two brothers, but not one, and that he would jump in to save eight cousins, but not seven.' The comment has become famous for it succinctly encapsulates the logic of inclusive fitness theory and its foundational assumption that as genetic relatedness decreases so does altruistic behaviour (Dugatkin 2007: 1376).

However, the concept of inclusive fitness has been critiqued by biologists who have noted the frequency of cooperation and altruism between individuals who are not genetically related. Such critiques are part of the broader 'levels of selection debate' (Okasha 2006: 143–69); for example, does natural selection act on the genes that individuals carry (along with copies of those genes carried by kin) or can it act upon larger biological entities such as groups of individuals who may not be genetically related? The possibility of the latter has led to the consideration of group selection theory as a possible means of explaining cooperation between unrelated individuals (Wilson and Wilson 2007).

The theoretical problem that inclusive fitness theory was unable to adequately deal with was the existence of altruistic acts and cooperation between non-kin. This undermined the assumption that evolutionary processes are characterised by a strong correlation between cooperation and genetic relatedness. As biologist E.O. Wilson writes inclusive fitness theory 'is a phantom mathematical construction that cannot be fixed in any manner that conveys realistic biological meaning. Nor can it be used to track the evolutionary dynamics of genetically based social systems' (Wilson 2012: 182). The key point to emphasise here is the need to explain the evolution of genetically based social systems, which as Wilson suggests inclusive fitness theory is unable to do.

In *Darwin's Cathedral*, Sloan Wilson applies the concept of group selection to the evolution of religion and the formation of moral communities. As Wilson writes, in moral communities 'social norms can create a degree of behavioural uniformity within groups and differences among groups that could never be predicted from their genetic structure and which is highly favourable for among-group selection' (Wilson 2003: 22). What Wilson is suggesting here is that social norms that prescribe sharing between unrelated members of a group can result in benefits that accrue to that group relative to social groups that lack such norms. The consequence is that evolutionary processes may favour groups that foster such norms. Consequently, the level at which natural selection is operating is not the individual, or the genes of individuals, but the social group.

What is significant about Wilson's approach to the evolution of religion and social groups is that he believes it to be compatible with Durkheim's conception of the social function of religion. As he writes, the 'similarity between' Durkheim's notion of beliefs and practices that unite individuals into a single moral community and the 'biological concept of human groups' as products of evolutionary processes is 'unmistakable.' As he elaborates 'in modern evolutionary terms, Durkheim interpreted religion as an adaptation that enables human groups to function as harmonious and coordinated units' (Wilson 2003: 54).

Wilson makes no mention of Jung in *Darwin's Cathedral*. However, his model that synthesises Durkheim and modern evolutionary theory can be fruitfully applied to Jung. In Chapter 1, I discussed the indebtedness of Jung to the French sociological tradition, as well as both Jung and Durkheim drawing on the same anthropological texts in their writings on sociality, kinship, ritual, and symbolism. In the context of that analysis the fit between Wilson's theory and analytical psychology becomes apparent. To recall Jung's comment above that exogamy, by virtue of including 'other groups' can result in the extension of 'the orderly cohesion of the tribe' (Jung 1983: 69–70). He also stated that the 'primitive system of marriage classes' are 'a vital necessity in the organization of the tribe' and that through the practice of 'exogamous marriage' the 'group acquires an inner stability, opportunities for expansion, and hence greater security.' Consequently, Jung argues that the 'main source of fear does not lie inside the group, but in the very real risks which the struggle for existence entail' (Jung 2014d: 327 and 233). Jung wrote these words long before the modern levels of selection debate and the development of models of group selection. However, it is clear that Jung is focussing on the evolutionary benefits of group-level adaptations. Consequently, there are important aspects of Jung's thinking that are consilient with modern theories of group and multilevel selection.

The other aspect of Wilson's model that is relevant to both Durkheim and Jung is the importance he places on symbols and ritual in bonding individuals into groups. In this sense ritual is an expression of the evolutionary process of group selection; as he writes:

> Durkheim felt that the symbolic badge of group membership and the aura of sacredness surrounding prescribed behaviours were required for clans to exist as functioning groups. He also felt that periodic gatherings were required to maintain the integrity of groups. The religious rituals and other festivities held during these gatherings were so emotionally intense that they gave force to group identity when its members were dispersed.
>
> (Wilson 2003: 54)

What I hope the above discussion makes clear is that there are unexplored aspects of Jung's work that not only show deep affinities with Durkheim and the French sociological tradition, but also contemporary evolutionary theory. I should add one caveat here; while I explore theories of how social cooperation may have evolved, I think there are certain aspects of ritual life that cannot be explained as adaptations. This is due to the fact that rituals seem to be specifically designed to disengage aspects of recently evolved neural architecture; that is, their purpose is to decrease activation in higher cortical centres while increasing activation in more ancient brain systems, a kind of phylogenetic regression if you like. Jung's concept of ritual as a very early form of psychotherapy offers a richer account of religious phenomenology than orthodox evolutionary or adaptationist accounts – for example, those developed by Wilson, Dunbar and Boyer to name a few (Wilson 2003; Boyer 2008; Dunbar 2014: 279–80, 2022). I explore these issues in more detail in Chapters 5 and 6.

In exploring the evolutionary origins of human cooperation and prosociality, fossil evidence can provide suggestive, but obviously not conclusive evidence for how it arose. In what follows, I explore various theories that have been proposed to explain human prosociality. This will involve an analysis of some of the most ancient hominin fossils. One of the theories I discuss is a variation on that outlined in Chapter 3 – that is, the exaptation of the neurobiology involved in the attachment between mothers and infants in adulthood social and sexual psychology. I will endeavour to connect this approach with group selection theory. Some researchers have argued that the exaptation of ancient maternal nurturant neurochemistry began very early in hominin evolution, millions of years before brain and body size increased and the associated cognitive capacity to make and utilise complex hunting technologies. In terms of Jungian theory, this would mean that our deep affective self, which serves as the archetypal basis of modern cognitive life, evolved millions of years before the emergence of ego consciousness.

The Miocene and Hominin Origins: Heterochrony and Life History Theory

It will be remembered from the discussion in Chapter 1 that Jung's evolutionary conception of the mind was based on his theory of an 'archaeologically layered psyche.' This theory was prompted by his dream of the successive layers or stories of a house, with the lowest layer containing skulls of *Pithecanthropus* (*Homo erectus*) and Neanderthals. As Jung elaborated on this conception of brain evolution:

> For just as a man has a body which is no different in principle from that of an animal, so also his psychology has a whole series of lower storeys in which the spectres from humanity's past epochs still dwell, then the animal souls from the age of Pithecanthropus and the hominids, then the "psyche" of the cold-blooded saurian.
>
> (Jung 1970: 212–3)

The term hominids generally refers to the Hominidae or great apes – which includes chimpanzees, bonobos, gorillas, orangutans and of all the hominin species in the lineage leading to modern humans. Elaborating on this idea, Jung also argued that the role 'consciousness plays in the life of … primates is insignificant compared with that of the unconscious' (Jung 2014b: 316). The implication of these comments is that the unconscious in contemporary humans is not just a product of past hominin evolution – but also the much more ancient evolution of primates.

What Jung is essentially arguing is that the primate period of our evolutionary history is still retained within the neurobiology of the modern human brain, but in a lower evolutionary layer of the brain. Elsewhere he extended the layer metaphor explicitly referring to our ancient primate heritage:

> We keep forgetting that we are primates and that we have to make allowances for these primitive layers in our psyche.
>
> (Jung 2020: 202)

When Jung wrote these words, we lacked information on the chronology of the transition from primate ancestor into hominins and then the evolution of modern humans or *Homo sapiens*. Current estimates based on both genetic and fossil evidence, suggest that hominins share a common ancestor with chimpanzees and bonobos approximately 6 to 7 million years ago and with gorillas 8 to 10 million years ago.

Throughout most of the twentieth century, it was assumed that early hominins evolved in open grass land and savanna habitats. However, in recent decades there has been accumulating evidence that many of our distinctive features, such as lack of large aggressive canine teeth and bipedal posture, evolved in forest and woodland habitats. Consequently, many researchers now argue that in order to understand hominin evolution, we need to go further back in time to the forest and woodland ecologies of the Miocene.

The Miocene is the period from 25 to 5 million years ago. During that period, Africa was much more densely forested than it is today. Many of the regions where fossils are found from the Miocene are now deserts – however, those habitats were once richly vegetated with an abundance of flora and fauna that have since become extinct due to a changing climate and the associated processes of deforestation and desertification. Some of the fossils from this period include the 7-million-year-old putative hominin *Sahelanthropus tchadensis*, which was discovered in the dry and inhospitable Djurab Desert in Chad – a region that 7 million years ago was rich in vegetation, woodland and river systems (Brunet et al. 2002). Another important fossil is *Ardipithecus kadabba*, a Miocene hominin dated at about five and half million years old (Haile-Selassie and WoldeGabriel 2009). *Ardipithecus kadabba* shows some of the first signs of reduction in canine morphology with the absence of a canine honing complex – a trait that signals the emergence of hominins (Haile-Selassie, Suwa, and White 2004).

In their book *The Ape in the Tree*, Alan Walker and Pat Shipman give some idea of the possible ecological context of social life for Miocene apes:

> Old World monkey species sometimes feed and travel in mixed species groups, recognize each other's alarm calls, and seem to benefit more than they are hurt by sharing their habitat with other species. Behavioural ecologists today know a good deal about how these varied monkeys partition up the forest and its resources, which allows them to co-exist without crippling competition. As we look at the Miocene sites in Africa, we see a similar pattern except that the fossil primates are early apes, not monkeys.
>
> (Walker and Shipman 2005: 9)

This is the ecological context that many researchers believe early hominins would have evolved in. The next geological epoch after the Miocene is the Pliocene, and it extends from 5 to 2 million years ago. The fascinating *Ardipithecus ramidus* fossils, which consist of the majority of a skeleton with hands, feet, pelvis and skull, have been dated to four and a half million years, which is the beginning of the Pliocene. During the early Pliocene, the ecological contexts were much the same as the Miocene, and like many Miocene apes *Ardipithecus ramidus* lived in a forest and woodland habitat. For example, while being partly bipedal, *Ardipithecus ramidus* also had feet with grasping big toes. In other primates feet with grasping big toes are used like a hand to climb trees. From this and other evidence it has been concluded that *Ardipithecus ramidus* inhabited the ancient forests of Pliocene Africa (Lovejoy et al. 2009).

The other fascinating feature of *Ardipithecus ramidus* is that it does not have large aggressive canines. In Figure 4.1, the contrast with chimpanzee canines is illustrated. As can be seen the chimpanzee has a large projecting face which houses what is called the canine honing complex. This morphological structure enables the upper canine to sharpen or hone on the lower premolar. It functions like a knife sharpener, ensuing the edge of the canine teeth are razor sharp. Chimpanzee males use these teeth in fights to establish dominance – and they can be deadly. Male chimpanzees have been known to disembowel their combatants with their aggressive canine armoury. As can be seen in Figure 4.1, the *Ardipithecus ramidus* skull is very much like a chimpanzee in terms of size and cranial capacity – but it lacks the projecting face and canine honing complex. The question paleoanthropologists seek to answer is why?

Some researchers have argued that the lack of aggressive canine armoury in *Ardipithecus ramidus* suggests this early hominin may have been less aggressive than other primates (Suwa et al. 2021). This is because sharp aggressive canines are the primary means by which primate males fight with one another to establish dominance. The absence of such canines so early in hominin evolution has led to the suggestion that males in this species may have contributed to infant and child development through provisioning mothers and their offspring (Lovejoy 2009). That is, in this species of early hominin, we see the evolutionary emergence of what eventually became fatherhood. Consequently, as opposed to expending reproductive effort on fighting other males, it would have been advantageous to begin provisioning mothers and their infants, with females preferring males who are so predisposed as mates. In this sense, more nurturing and cooperative males would

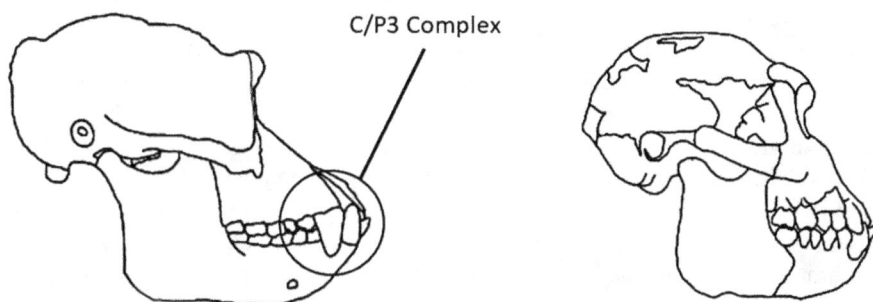

Figure 4.1 This figure illustrates the C/P3 or canine honing complex. On the left, a chimpanzee; on the right, the early hominin *Ardipithecus ramidus*. In the chimpanzee, the upper canine hones or sharpens against the lower premolar. This honing complex is absent in *Ardipithecus ramidus*. See text for details. Adapted from Clark and Henneberg (2017).

have gained an evolutionary advantage through female mate selection (Clark and Henneberg 2015). This thesis also postulates that the brains of *Ardipithecus ramidus* males may have had upregulated oxytocin levels as we find in the males of other mammal species who engage in infant and child care – including our own (Lovejoy 2009).

These theories of course are speculative. But they are based on comparative data and how that data can be used to predict the social and sexual psychology of ancient hominin species (Lovejoy 2009). Importantly, very early in hominin evolution we begin to see the 'feminisation' of male skull and canine morphology – that is, male hominins come to resemble the females of other primates such as chimpanzees more than they do the males. *Ardipithecus ramidus* is one of the earliest examples we have of such feminisation (Suwa et al. 2009; White, Suwa, and Lovejoy 2010). Importantly, feminisation of male morphology also results in a reduction in the differences between male and female canine size – that is, reduced canine sexual dimorphism.

There are some very suggestive observations here when thinking about analytical psychology and particularly Jung's theory of a feminine component in the male psyche. The research cited above makes two claims: that the skull and canine morphology of early hominin males became feminised and less aggressive and that accompanying this change there was also an upregulation of female mammalian nurturant neurochemicals such as oxytocin in the male brain. This may be the deep evolutionary origins of the anima – that is, a feminine component in the deeper unconscious layers of the male brain.

Of course, we can never be certain about these issues, and other researchers propose different scenarios about the evolution of hominin sociality. For example, some researchers argue against reduced sexual dimorphism in early hominin evolution and that the latter group of hominins such as the Australopithecines, which emerge some three and a half million years ago, were extremely sexually dimorphic and unlike humans – while other researchers found reduced sexual dimorphism in this group (Reno et al. 2003; Gordon 2013; Reno and Lovejoy 2015). It has also been argued that early hominin social and familial structure was similar to the high sexually dimorphic gorilla, with a large dominant male silverback and a harem of much smaller females (Geary and Flinn 2001).

This debate will no doubt continue for some time to come. What is clear however is that the large aggressive canines characteristic of other male primates is absent in the earliest hominin species. And if as it has been argued, mammalian nurturant neurochemicals were upregulated in the male brain of early hominins such as *Ardipithecus ramidus*, then this would mean a very early emergence of what Jung called the anima – the feminine counterpart in the male brain.

What is significant about *Ardipithecus ramidus* is that while it lacks large aggressive canine armoury, it still has a brain about the same size as a chimpanzee. What this implies is that hominin social behaviour, and the trend towards higher levels of cooperation, evolved long before hominin brain and body size increased among *Homo erectus*, which emerged during the Pleistocene some 2 million years after *Ardipithecus ramidus*. Brain size is also important for reconstructing the ontogeny of extinct hominins. No direct evidence of ontogeny or brain development exists but we can predict developmental trajectories from brain size. This is because brain size correlates with developmental trajectories in primates. This makes sense – it takes longer to grow a larger brain and body which means as a general principle animals with larger brains will reach sexual maturity later than animals with smaller brains.

The most significant among these correlations is that brain size is correlated with the age of first birth across primates species (Smith and Tompkins 1995). The equations for these correlations can then be used to predict the ontogeny of extinct hominins – given we know the brain size from the skulls we can predict trajectories of development. In our own research on *Ardipithecus ramidus* we concluded that this species matured at about the same rate as chimpanzees – which is to be expected given it has a brain size similar to chimpanzees. However, the ontogeny of craniofacial and canine maturation seems to have been retarded relative chimpanzees (Clark and Henneberg 2015, 2017).

This can be seen in Figure 4.1 where the chimpanzee face and canines project much more than in *Ardipithecus ramidus*; yet, both species have a cranium, and hence a brain, of similar size. Based on the above equations, we argued that *Ardipithecus ramidus* most likely reached sexual maturity around the same age as chimpanzees – but that growth in the facial region that houses the canines as well as the growth of the canines themselves were developmentally retarded. We interpreted these findings in terms of Haeckel's concept of heterochrony where growth in different ontogenetic fields could be altered in relation to one another (Clark and Henneberg 2015). That is, relative to chimpanzees and the last common ancestor, maturational rates did not change but the anatomy of the face, jaw and canines did. This is an example of Kant's theory of speciation discussed in Chapter 1; as he wrote 'the proliferation of species might arise according to a simple outline: the shortening of one part or the lengthening of another, the development of one part or the atrophy of another' (Kant quoted in Richards 2000: 28). In *Ardipithecus ramidus*, we see shortening or reduced growth of the canines and the regions in the face and jaw that house them. However brain size – and most likely the associated ontogenetic trajectories – remained pretty much the same as chimpanzees and bonobos. Consequently, brain size and maturational rates were retained from the Miocene common ancestor hominins share with chimpanzees and bonobos – while the face, jaw and canine morphology were reduced or to use Kant's terminology shortened or atrophied.

Human ontogeny is delayed relative to chimpanzees mainly because it takes longer for our larger brains and bodies to develop. This contrast can be seen in Figure 4.2 which illustrates the different ontogenetic trajectories evident when comparing humans with chimpanzees. For example, after birth and during the first of year life, chimpanzee brain growth tails off. However, in humans the brain continues to grow until about the age of five or six. Additionally, humans reach sexual maturity some five to six years later than chimpanzees and bonobos (Bogin 2003; Clark and

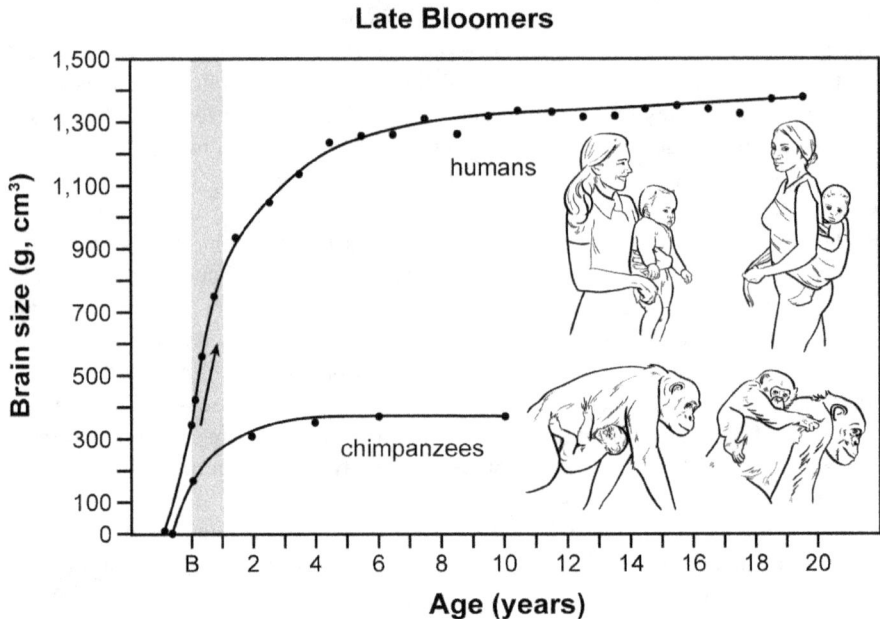

Figure 4.2 This figure illustrates the different developmental trajectories of chimpanzee and human brain growth. See text for details. From Falk (2016). With permission from the author.

Henneberg 2015). For example, chimpanzees begin reproducing around eight years of age with the average age of first birth being about 11 years of age, whereas for human females, sexual maturity is delayed and average age of reproduction is 19 years (Lathouwers and Elsacker 2005; Clark and Henneberg 2015).

This extension of ontogeny relative to other primates, means that humans have delayed schedules of dental eruption, cessation of brain development and delayed onset of sexual maturation (Minugh-Purvis and McNamara 2002; Hawkes and Paine 2006; Trevathan and Rosenberg 2016). This unique ontogenetic trajectory results in humans having extended periods of development that we refer to as childhood and adolescence. These periods of growth are necessary for the development of our unique linguistic and socio-cognitive capacities and it is one of the central developmental features that distinguish humans from other primates (Bogin and Smith 1996; Bogin 2003; Locke and Bogin 2006; Falk 2016; Clark and Henneberg 2017). Importantly, it is during the adolescent period of growth that we see maturation of the default mode network, a uniquely human neural hub associated with complex social cognition and the emergence of a sense of self or ego consciousness (Carhart-Harris and Friston 2010; Clark 2022). During the adolescent period of development, we also see a transition from primary to secondary consciousness – that is, from subcortical to more cortical control of behaviour (Fair et al. 2008; Jones 2013).

The crucial issue when understanding early hominins such as *Ardipithecus ramidus* is that like chimpanzees and bonobos, given similar brain size, this species would have lacked the extended ontogeny characteristic of modern humans (Clark and Henneberg 2015, 2017). However, based on the reduction in canines, it would have mostly evolved very different forms of social and sexual psychology compared with bonbons and chimpanzees.

The important point to emphasise about the above discussion is that the extension of life history or slowed maturation associated with our unique form of consciousness is an example of the relationship between ontogeny and phylogeny. For example, in order for humans to develop their unique form of consciousness required a change in ontogenetic growth trajectories associated with brain maturation. This change was from a maturational schedule like that of a chimpanzee or early hominin like *Ardipithecus ramidus*, to one similar to our own, with an adolescent period of growth and delayed onset of sexual maturation. In this sense, cognitive phylogenesis seems to have occurred through the evolution of ontogeny. Or as Brain Hall has expressed the notion: ontogeny does not recapitulate phylogeny; it creates phylogeny (Hall 2011).

With these observations in mind, let us return to Jung's conception of the evolution of consciousness:

Consciousness is phylogenetically and ontogenetically a secondary phenomenon. It is time this obvious fact were grasped at last. Just as the body has an anatomical prehistory of millions of years, so also does the psychic system. And just as the human body today represents in each of its parts the result of this evolution, and everywhere still shows traces of its earlier stages so the same may be said of the psyche. Consciousness began its evolution from an animal-like state which seems to us unconscious, and the same process of differentiation is repeated in every child.

(Jung 2011: 348)

We can see here that Jung is not arguing that our ancestors were the mental equivalent of children as has been suggested in regard to his use of Haeckel's biogenetic law (Otis 1994: 208). What he is suggesting is that in both phylogeny and ontogeny, consciousness is a secondary phenomenon that developed after and upon an antecedent system of foundational unconscious brain process – or what he has referred to elsewhere as subcortical affect-based brain systems (Jung 1960: 170–1).

We can add to and refine Jung's theory of the phylogenesis of consciousness in light of current research. For example, his assertion that consciousness began its 'evolution from an animal-like state which seems to us unconscious, and the same process of differentiation is repeated in every child' can be interpreted from the point of view of life history theory discussed above. For example, for early hominins such as *Ardipithecus ramidus* with an ontogeny like chimpanzees, we could consider to be existing in the 'animal-like state' – or what we might call a primary process socio-affective mode. In order for consciousness to emerge over evolutionary time, this chimpanzee-like ontogeny would need to be extended into one with a longer period of brain maturation eventually resulting in an adolescent period of growth. The result of such an extension would be a transition from primary consciousness to a form of secondary consciousness with the associated default mode network and ego functions. And here is the important point: each child as they mature retraces that trajectory from primary process to secondary process during ontogeny. But the only reason a modern child has a delayed ontogeny is because ontogeny was delayed over evolutionary time – that is, during phylogeny.

The above approach is one of the many examples of the relationship between ontogeny and phylogeny developed by Haeckel. It is not so much an example of recapitulation as early hominins were not the equivalent of modern children – they were fully grown adults with mature morphology that had developed past the childhood phase not remained at it. The relationship between ontogeny and phylogeny outlined above is an example of what Haeckel called heterochrony – that is, alteration of the developmental timing of growth trajectories in descendent species in relation to their ancestors. The heterochronic alteration of ontogenetic trajectories from early hominins like *Ardipithecus ramidus* to modern humans like ourselves involved delayed neural and sexual maturation with the consequent evolution of an adolescent period of growth. It is this extension of ontogeny over evolutionary time that seems to have given rise to what Jung referred to as the conscious ego (Clark 2022).

Homo erectus and Neanderthals: Life History and the Evolution of Adolescence

One of the major changes in human evolution is the increase in brain and body size during the Pleistocene. The Pleistocene is the period from 2 million to 10,000 years ago. These increases in brain and body size first appear during the early Pleistocene with the emergence of *Homo erectus*. Additionally, not only do we see larger brains and bodies that begin to resemble modern humans during this period, we also see increasing evidence of hunting, more complex technologies and social complexity. Numerous researchers argue that such technical and social developments required an extended period of brain development and socialisation during which the elderly could teach the young increasingly complex skills such as tool manufacture (Sterelny 2012). The implication is that *Homo erectus* had an ontogeny markedly different from earlier hominins such as *Ardipithecus ramidus* and the Australopithecines. Based on the above mentioned correlations between brain size and maturational rates, it seems that an extended period of brain maturation may have first emerged among *Homo erectus* some 2 million years ago.

The above analysis is based on research that has taken place since the 1990s. The field of palaeoanthropology was in its infancy when Jung was alive and many of the hypotheses of that period are no longer accepted by contemporary researchers. One of the commonly held views in the first half of the twentieth century was that *Homo erectus* and Neanderthals were vastly different creatures from modern humans, being intermediate ape-like creatures between *Homo sapiens* and the other great apes. This was the view held by Jung. Current research places both groups much closer to humans than apes, with some even arguing that they may be populational variants of our own lineage, and in that sense very much human like ourselves. A modern form of analytical psychology informed by contemporary evolutionary theory would need to take these issues into account and update Jung's views accordingly.

To recall Jung's comment on Dubois' Pithecanthropus (*Homo erectus*) fossil where he stated that the human psyche possesses 'a whole series of lower storeys in which the spectres from humanity's past epochs still dwell, then the animal souls from the age of Pithecanthropus and the hominids' (Jung 1970: 212–3). In Jung's comment, he seems to be associating Pithecanthropus with the other apes. He makes this association explicit when contrasting the supposed psychology of *Homo erectus* and Neanderthals with modern humans. As he writes, 'Sinanthropos man' (another *Homo erectus* fossil) and 'the Neanderthal race ... are immensely old, because the anatomical features have changed considerably since.' Jung goes on to contrast the psychology of these early varieties of hominin – what he designates the 'old man' or 'ape man' – with modern forms of consciousness (Jung 1998: 1194–5).

Pithecanthropus erectus was the name given to a skull found in 1891 on the island of Java in Indonesia by the Dutch paleoanthropologist Eugene Dubois (1858–1940). The name *Pithecanthropus erectus* ('upright ape-man') is derived from the Latin pithec for ape and anthropos for human, with erectus signifying upright or bipedal posture. This taxonomic classification characterised the fossil as not only a different species than ourselves, but as an entirely different genus. This taxonomic distinction was based on Dubois' belief that *Pithecanthropus erectus* was an 'intermediate being between humans and apes' (Cela-Conde and Ayala 2007: 88). Dubois' taxonomic classification was later revised in the 1950s as the degree of difference between *Homo erectus* and *Homo sapiens* is not sufficient to justify the recognition of *Pithecanthropus* as a separate genus (Mayr 1963: 341).

Since Dubois's discovery many more fossils have been found that show similarities with *Pithecanthropus*. In modern taxonomic nomenclature they are collectively known as *Homo erectus* with the first examples of the group emerging in Africa approximately 2 million years ago (Herries et al. 2020). Members of the *Homo erectus* group had migrated to Europe and reached Asia by half a million years ago if not earlier (Zhou et al. 2000).

It is unclear if *Homo erectus* possessed an ontogeny similar to *Homo sapiens* with the slowed maturation rates and an adolescent period of socio-cognitive development of the kind that characterises our species. Some research indicates that the ontogeny of *Homo erectus* was unique, with the modern developmental pattern occurring quite late in hominin evolution (Dean and Smith 2009; Dean et al. 2001) and possibly emerging with the evolution of *Homo sapiens* (Bogin 2003). Hublin and colleagues adopt this approach, arguing that the modern life history pattern emerged in the last 'few hundred thousand years along the evolutionary line leading to extant modern humans.' Elaborating on this perspective and the implications for hominin brain ontogeny they argue that the 'life-history pattern and brain ontogeny of extant humans emerged only recently in the course of human evolution' (Hublin, Neubauer, and Gunz 2015: 8 and 1).

Other researchers, however, have argued the life history pattern of *Homo erectus* and *Homo sapiens* were similar (Antón and Leigh 2003) and that an adolescent stage of development may have evolved in later *Homo erectus* during the middle Pleistocene as 'life histories near those of living humans would be expected to arise as [hominin] brain size crested 1000 cc' (Smith and Tompkins 1995: 264). In addition to this evidence based on correlations between brain size and ontogeny, work looking at variation in dental development in modern humans suggests that early *Homo* tooth formation does in fact lie within the range modern humans (Dean and Liversidge 2015; Xing et al. 2019). Further evidence for such affinities comes from the fossils found at the Xujiayao site in China. These fossils, which may be as old as 200,000 years, represent a combination of archaic *Homo erectus* with more modern *Homo sapiens* features. Significantly, one of the juvenile specimens seems to have a pattern of dental development similar to modern humans, leading researchers to conclude that 'modern human dental growth and development evolved in East Asia before the appearance of fully modern human morphology' (Xing et al. 2019: 1).

Other evidence that a modern life history pattern and brain ontogeny existed in *Homo erectus* comes from the archaeological record. Among *Homo erectus* deposits, we begin to see associated tool technologies such as Acheulean tools. Acheulean tools seem to have emerged approximately 2 million years ago. They are complex symmetrical tools that are still used by contemporary hunter-gatherers primarily for cutting or as spear heads. Reflecting on the similar technologies used by *Homo erectus* and modern humans, it has been argued that '… past and modern humans share a common body structure and the same physical constraints' and that consequently the uniformity 'between current and extinct populations can provide a fundamental way of understanding manufacture technologies of stone tools from all periods' (Chen and Chen 2016: 93). Significantly, the ability to learn the skills necessary to manufacture complex Acheulean technologies of the kind *Homo erectus* is presumed to have made, most likely required an extended life history akin to modern humans with a childhood and adolescent period of socio-cognitive development – that is a period of apprenticeship during which culturally accumulated technical knowledge is transferred from one generation to the next (Sterelny 2012).

Acheulean tools are complex symmetrical objects. Their makers would have been capable of internal cognitive representations enabling them to preconceive, plan and execute the multiple steps necessary to make such objects. Acheulean tools are also believed to require cognitive representations such as 'projective and euclidean spatial operations' (Wynn 1989: 89–90). Significantly, fMRI studies have suggested Acheulean toolmaking, in contrast to the much older and rudimentary non-symmetrical Oldowan technologies, recruits brain regions associated with the default mode network, planning, learning, social scaffolding, 'central executive' working memory and 'mental time travel' (Stout et al. 2015). Significantly, mental time travel, which involves the projection of the self into both past and future scenarios, is believed to be fundamental to the hunter-gatherer adaptation that led to the demographic expansion of the genus *Homo* out of Africa and into China some 2 million years ago (Corballis 2019). Given the default mode network is believed to be associated with secondary consciousness, and the emergence of an enduring sense of self or ego (Carhart-Harris and Friston 2010), it seems possible that such a mode of consciousness may have been present in *Homo erectus*.

With Neanderthals, the evidence of a close evolutionary relationship with modern humans is much stronger than in *Homo erectus*. This is mainly because researchers have been able to extract genetic material from Neanderthal fossils. These studies in paleogenomics have found that modern humans contain between 1 and 4 per cent Neanderthal DNA (Pääbo 2014). The consequences of these findings is that it is unlikely Neanderthals are a separate species as interbreeding and producing viable offspring are usually considered criteria for being the same species. Given our ancestors must have bred with Neanderthals, it is most likely they were not a separate species but a populational variant within our lineage that *Homo sapiens* could breed with and produce viable offspring with (Prüfer et al. 2014).

Other evidence of affinities between ourselves and Neanderthals comes from an increasingly rich archaeological record. For example, evidence of the use of ochre by Neanderthals 200,000 years ago (Roebroeks et al. 2012) as well as ochre applied to perforated marine shells around 120,000 years ago (Hoffmann et al. 2018) has led to an appreciation of possible forms of symbolic culture in this group of hominins. Additionally, it has been argued that symbolic culture, body ornamentation and jewellery in Neanderthal deposits indicates modern forms of culture and that the differences between Neanderthals and modern humans is cultural and not genetic or cognitively based (Arsuaga 2009; Zilhão et al. 2010).

There is also evidence from caves in France of Neanderthals creating geometric structures made of stalagmites and that consequently social organisation among this group of hominin was most likely more complex than previously thought (Jaubert et al. 2016). Additionally, Neanderthals are believed to have made and used musical instruments – abilities that were once thought to be unique to *Homo sapiens* (Turk et al. 2018). While nothing is ever certain in archaeology and palaeoanthropology, and new discoveries are likely to undermine current theories, there is a significant body of evidence suggesting that Neanderthals were fully human, possessing minds, emotions and spiritual beliefs similar to our own (Arsuaga 2009).

The above discussion suggests that if *Ardipithecus ramidus*, and other small-brained hominins such as the Australopithecines, matured at about the same rate as chimpanzees, it is unlikely that they developed a modern form of the default mode network and the associated forms of ego consciousness and sense of self – which as noted above require an extended period of growth and adolescent development before reaching adulthood. In more recent species such as *Homo erectus* (Jung's *Pithecanthropus*), that network may have started to develop the capacities we find in modern humans (Clark and Henneberg 2021a) which include metacognition, mental time, internal rumination as well as the formation of a sense of self or ego consciousness (Carhart-Harris and Friston 2010; Clark 2022).

Consequently, we may reconceptualise Jung's 'primate layer' in the psyche in terms of Miocene apes and early ape-like hominins such as *Ardipithecus ramidus*. His designation of Neanderthals and *Homo erectus* as varieties of 'ape man' is not a view supported by the evidence that has accumulated since his passing. In our research, we concluded that most of the major components of human cognition and social psychology were already in place in *Homo erectus* – a view based on complex tool technologies as well as the putative manufacture and navigation of marine craft by *Homo erectus* (Bednarik 2015; Clark and Henneberg 2021a, 2021b). My suspicion is if a young *Homo erectus* child were raised in our culture, they could probably quite easily learn how to use a computer or fix car engines. However, this is a controversial view, and others argue that modern human cognition has a much more recent origin (Hare 2017; Benítez-Burraco and Kempe 2018). What seems to be clear is that *Homo erectus* and Neanderthals are more closely related to modern humans than Jung thought when he referred to them as examples of 'ape-man.' How closely related however is still a point of contention in palaeoanthropology.

The Archaeology of Mind and Cross-Species Homologies: Ancient Jewels and Treasures

It will be recalled from Chapter 1 that evolutionary biologists refer to shared anatomical features in distantly related species as homologies. In that discussion I noted how this concept was derived from the *Naturphilosophen's* concept of anatomical archetypes and developed by the English palaeontologist Richard Owen (1804–1892) in works such as *On the Archetype and Homologies of the Vertebrate Skeleton* (1848). Owen's theories were important for Darwin who interpreted archetypes as ancestors, with descent from a common ancestor providing the explanation for archetypal or homologous structures (Hall 1993: 58). It is this tradition, from the *Naturphilosophen* through to Haeckel and Darwin, that informs Jung's concept of deep affinities between ourselves and our hominin and primate ancestors.

While Jung did not use the concept of homology, his theory of archetypes is essentially describing homologous structures in the brain that modern humans share with not only ancient hominins but also other species. If we find similar structures or neurobiological substrates in widely separated species – for example, mice, elephants and humans – the most parsimonious explanation is that such structures existed in the common ancestor of all three animals. This is not always the case – similar structures can evolve independently in different taxonomic groups through convergent evolution. But as a general rule when a number of species share similar anatomical structures or neurobiology, it is likely those species had a common ancestor in their distant evolutionary past who possessed those traits. Additionally, if we find large numbers of species possessing the same traits, this provides further evidence for a common ancestry.

Mammals are an example of a taxonomic group with shared homologous structures – particularly in the neurobiology of attachment and social bonding. I already explored these issues in Chapter 2 in relation to the oxytocin system. In what follows, I extend that analysis in a discussion of different theories which seek to explain the evolution of human cooperation. In this sense I will be addressing the levels of selection debate and Durkheim's theory about the evolution of cooperation discussed earlier in this chapter – and Jung's focus on the same issue in his writings about group-level cooperation.

There are two main theories in human evolutionary studies that seek to explain the evolution of cooperation, altruism and empathy. One postulates that conflict between closed social groups led to selection for groups with more cooperative individuals. This theory is predicted on the assumption that conflict between groups has been a consistent feature of human evolution over hundreds of thousands if not millions of years. This approach is a variation on the group selection hypothesis discussed above. The other theory postulates the exaptation of very ancient and homologous (what Jung would call archetypal) neurobiology for uses other than those for which it evolved. These homologous systems are the neurobiology of mammalian nurturant behaviour that facilitates bonding between mothers and offspring. In this model, human empathy, altruism and cooperation result from the exaptation of this ancient neurobiological substrate in adulthood social and sexual psychology.

These two theories are not mutually exclusive. For example, some species such as chimpanzees utilise the oxytocin system to establish bonds between individuals before they engage in conflict with another group (Samuni et al. 2017). But this does not mean that the oxytocin system evolved for this purpose – it means that it has most likely been exapted or repurposed for intergroup conflict. It may be reinforced by natural selection if the behaviours benefit the survival of the group and the individuals who are members of that group. But such selection on pre-existent structures means current use is not the same as evolutionary origin. A correlate of this position is that such pre-existent structures can have a number of current, and often vastly different, uses among extant species. As we will see, this is the case in chimpanzees and bonobos – species that utilise the oxytocin system in dramatically different and species-specific ways.

The metaphor of an archeologically layered brain comprising homologous structures we share with other animals is one adopted by Jaak Panksepp in *The Archaeology of Mind: Neuroevolutionary Origins of Human Emotions*, written in collaboration with Lucy Biven. This model, in terms of both its scientific basis and the metaphors used, is very similar to Jung's conception of an archaeologically layered psyche discussed in Chapter 2.

These homologous structures, according to Panksepp and Biven, enable us to better understand the deep evolutionary origins of human emotion. As they write: '… it is now clear that animal models can promote an accurate archaeology of many of those ancient affective principles that still control human lives' (Panksepp and Biven 2012: 450). Such an approach seeks to understand the ancient emotional brain systems that evolved prior to the emergence of more complex forms of conscious learning associated with the neocortex. As they write, such an approach

> ... seeks to illuminate how our most powerful emotional feelings—the primal emotional affects—arise from ancient neural networks situated in brain regions below the neocortical "thinking-cap." The neocortex is an organ that generates complex cognitive abilities as well as culture, and it is definitively important for complex perceptions, learning, and cognitions. The neocortex is responsible for almost all of the cultural milestones that human beings have been able to achieve ... [T]he cortex could achieve nothing without an evolved foundational mind deeper in the brain. Those ancient neural territories below the neocortex constitute our ancestral mind—the affective mind, which is evolutionarily specialized and that we share with many other animals. It is "archaeological treasure," for it contains the sources of some of our most powerful feelings. Those ancient subcortical brain systems are precious, multihued "jewels" for anyone wishing to understand the roots of all the basic values we have ever known and will experience in our lives. The affects are the foundations upon which the beauty and ugliness of life has been constructed.
>
> (Panksepp and Biven 2012: x)

What is significant about their approach is the delineation of homologous brain regions and neurochemicals associated with maternal care. In this sense once this system was established in very early mammals it was conserved and maintained throughout the various diversifications of mammalian, primate and hominin lineages. As they write, commenting on the 'same symphony of maternal chemicals' that promotes offspring care across multiple mammalian species: '... given the homology of mammalian emotional systems, and given that all mammals, including our own species, universally exhibit maternal behaviours (with abundant differences in details among species), it is very likely that similar principles are at work in the brains of all mammals' (Panksepp and Biven 2012: 183). Significantly, Jung referred to 'big dreams' that emerge from the deeper evolutionary layers of the psyche as the 'richest jewel in the treasure-house of psychic experience' (Jung 2014c). Jung and Panksepp have, independently it seems, developed similar metaphors of an archeologically layered psyche in which jewels and treasures are discoverable in the deepest phylogenetically ancient regions of the brain – for Jung they are archetypal structures for Panksepp cross-species homologies. As my historical analysis in Chapter 1 indicated, the concept of homology was derived originally from the *Naturphilosophen* and the theory of anatomical archetypes that can be traced back to Goethe and Kant, and which via Owen informed Darwin's theory of shared ancestral forms. In much of Panksepp's discussion, the concept of homology could be replaced with archetypes without any real loss of meaning.

In Chapter 3, I discussed Panksepp's view that modern neuroscience provides some support for the Freudian view of a relationship between maternal attachment and adulthood sexuality. This view was based on the observation that neural systems for both forms of bonding are intermeshed in limbic areas of the brain. Panksepp argued that neuroscience has revealed the ancient 'neurosymbolic processes that first led to nurturance and social attachments in the mammalian brain' – processes which have important implications for the 'biological sources of friendship and love' (Panksepp 2004: 246). These homologous – or archetypal – brain structures we share with other mammals and which underpin maternal care can illuminate Bachofen's thesis discussed in Chapter 1 that 'the relationship which stands at the origin of all culture, of every virtue, of every nobler aspect of existence, is that between mother and child' (Bachofen 1967: 79). Reflecting on the affinities between the neurochemical pathways underpinning infant care and adulthood sociality, Patricia Churchland echoes Bachofen's theory when she avers that the 'extension of caring to dependent infants, and then to mates, kin, and affiliates, marks the crucial shift that makes us social' (Churchland 2018: 63).

The above outlines a model of the evolution of human cooperation, altruism and empathy based on exaptation of ancient homologous brain structures and neurochemistry we share with other mammals and primates. Stephanie Preston adopts a similar approach in her article 'The origins of altruism in offspring care' and in her book *The Altruistic Urge: Why We're Driven to Help Others* (Preston 2013, 2022). As Preston avers altruistic responding is facilitated by 'cues of target vulnerability, neoteny, distress, and a social bond—features that are all characteristic of contexts that involve caregiving and targets in genuine need.' She also argues that such responding in humans was extended from vulnerable neotenous infants to the broader social group resulting in a 'homology between offspring retrieval and primitive altruistic responding.' As she elaborates:

> … [in] human evolution, these active altruistic responses were likely further augmented and extended to include strategic forms of helping, sharing, and co-operation in larger group contexts where there existed additional pressures to maintain a reputation and compete for resources. Through such a stepwise process, all existing views on the evolution of altruism can be accommodated into one larger picture, which builds later forms of altruism upon the primitive base.
>
> (Preston 2013: 1328)

Examples of exaptation of the oxytocin system exist in humans, bonobos and chimpanzees. In both bonobos and chimpanzees, the oxytocin system is involved in group cohesion – but it functions in species-specific ways. For example, in chimpanzees, the oxytocin system seems to be associated with chimpanzee intergroup aggression, while in bonobos, it seems to facilitate both in-group cohesion and affiliative behaviour between groups (Brooks et al. 2022).

Chimpanzees are highly territorial and often engage in lethal violence with neighbouring groups using their canines as weapons to wound, disembowel or kill. Yet, such fighting requires individuals within the group to be tightly bonded in order to defeat the neighbouring group. It is believed that such ingroup cohesion exists in chimpanzees as a result of such intergroup conflict as well as predation pressure from leopards (Boesch 2009). Significantly, before engaging in an attack members of the group may groom one another in order to facilitate bonding which is associated with elevated levels of oxytocin. This parallels the function of oxytocin in humans where it increases in group cohesion in the face of external threat (Samuni et al. 2017).

Bonobos are very different in their social behaviour than chimpanzees, and they have not been reported to engage in lethal violence nor do groups engage in conflict. When groups meet as opposed to fighting, as in the case of chimpanzees, bonobo groups often merge, with the females from each group engaging in sex. It has been suggested that bonobos have a 'regional society above the group level' (Itani 1990: 153) in which groups forage 'together for as long as a week' (Hashimoto et al. 2008: 117). It is believed that such 'neighbourhood relations' facilitate a form of 'peaceful coexistence of two unit-groups' that parallels human sociality (Itani 1990: 184). This observation echoes Walker's comments quoted above that Miocene apes, like Old World monkeys, may have fed together and travelled in mixed species groups, allowing them to co-exist without crippling competition.

Significantly, when bonobo groups meet and establish such friendly relations, oxytocin levels are elevated – but not to bond the group so it can fight a neighbouring group but so that neighbouring groups can themselves bond. In this sense the oxytocin system can be exapted in species-specific ways, for in bonobos it is not associated with intergroup conflict but forms the physiological basis for increased motivation to cooperate and intergroup affiliation (Moscovice et al. 2019). Significantly, as already noted early hominins like *Ardipithecus ramidus* lack the aggressive canine and facial morphology of chimpanzees – they also show more affinity with the less aggressive morphology of bonobos (Suwa et al. 2009; Clark and Henneberg 2015). It has also been argued that reduced aggression, elevated levels of prosociality and possible alloparenting may have been facilitated by elevated levels of oxytocin in *Ardipithecus ramidus* (Lovejoy 2009; Clark and Henneberg 2017).

It is possible that the similarities between *Ardipithecus ramidus* and bonobo morphology are related to feeding ecology and resource availability. For example, chimpanzee habitats have been subject to climate change over the last 2 million years, while bonobo habitats have not. As a result, there is less competition for food among bonobos and consequently less conflict. More available food also means female bonobos can forage together, whereas female chimpanzees tend to forage alone as fruit in their habitats is more widely dispersed. If females can forage in groups, this is obviously beneficial if they need to form an alliance against males – which may be the reason why bonobo society is matriarchal or dominated by groups of females (Furuichi and Thompson 2007). Significantly, bonobo habitats and those of *Ardipithecus ramidus* most likely resemble those of Miocene Africa described by Walker more than chimpanzee habitats do.

Numerous researchers have argued that human cooperation evolved due to cooperative groups being able to out compete non-cooperative groups. This approach assumes that conflict between groups, in a manner similar to chimpanzees, is what led to the evolution of altruism, morality and group-level cooperation. From this perspective, lethal conflict between groups – that is, the evolutionary basis of warfare – is something that is very ancient and can be traced back to the common ancestor humans share with chimpanzees some 6 to 7 million years ago. Based on this model, E.O. Wilson has argued that intergroup conflict in our species is 'our hereditary curse' (Wilson 2012: 62). Jared Diamond has adopted a similar perspective extrapolating from chimpanzee lethal violence: 'of all our human landmarks – art, spoken language, drugs, and the others – the one that has been derived most straightforwardly from animal precursors is genocide' (Diamond 2006: 294).

The above theories have become known as the chimpanzee referential model in which chimpanzees are believed to provide a model for early hominin social life. With more recent fossil finds such as *Ardipithecus ramidus* which shows very few similarities with chimpanzees, this approach has been increasingly called into question (Sayers, Raghanti, and Lovejoy 2012; White et al. 2015; Clark and Henneberg 2015, 2017). These theorists propose other means by which cooperation could have evolved such as female sexual selection of more cooperative males, which would benefit males predisposed to share food and provision females and offspring. When species cooperate in this manner in the raising of offspring, it often scales up to more generalised social cooperation, possibly subserved by oxytocin and similar neurobiological substrates. In contrast to Wilson and Diamond, these approaches do not assume that human morality and cooperation evolved in a crucible of bloodshed and slaughter in which more cooperative groups committed acts of war and genocide against less cooperative groups.

To return to the issue of human sociality, cooperation and religion discussed at the start of this chapter when considering Durkheim's theories. In that section I discussed David Sloan-Wilson's *Darwin's Cathedral* and his argument that group selection had underpinned the evolution of religion. In that analysis he offered an evolutionary explanation for Durkheim's theories – and there I also suggested such an approach is useful when thinking about Jung's ideas on social evolution and the 'orderly cohesion of the tribe' (Jung 1983: 69–70).

Importantly, Jung believed that the forms of social libido that underpin religious cohesion have their basis in prior forms of parental attachment; as he writes the 'benefits of religion are equivalent in their effects, to the parental care lavished upon the child' going on to state that 'religious feelings are rooted in unconscious memories of certain tender emotions in early infancy' which Jung refers to as 'memories of archetypal intuitions' (Jung 2014d: 89). This view of human sociality is very much the same as that proposed by Panksepp and Preston in which adult social psychology is subserved by primal neurobiological systems that originally evolved to facilitate attachment between mothers and infants. Where they differ from Jung is they were able to ground their ideas in ancient homologous (archetypal) neurobiological substrates and neurochemistry. If Jung were alive today, he very well likely would have refined his thinking based on these findings in modern evolutionary neuroscience which support some of his central contentions.

As already noted the oxytocin system subserves sexual bonding (Light, Grewen, and Amico 2005; Panksepp and Biven 2012: 241) parental psychology

(Gordon et al. 2010) as well as generalised cooperation (Rilling et al. 2012). It is also involved in the social dimensions of music, such as trust and cooperation within groups of culturally compatible but not necessarily genetically related individuals – aspects of sociality that are believed to stimulate reward and motivation due to music's impact on the limbic system (Harvey 2020). Dance also induces pleasurable arousal and positive prosocial mood via the release of endorphins and neurohormones such as oxytocin (Laland, Wilkins, and Clayton 2016).

Based on these findings it has been argued that human ritual and dance seem to have exapted maternal neurobiology and the oxytocin system to facilitate bonding between adults (Dissanayake 2021). Consequently, it seems likely that the forms of cooperation, social bonding and group ritual analysed by both Durkheim and Jung exploit this ancient system. It also means that social cooperation, bonding and empathy may be used in group-level conflict – but it does not mean such emotions necessarily evolved in our lineage because of group-level conflict. In other words, the neurobiological substrates of social cooperation, bonding and empathy can be utilised in any number of contexts – only one of which is conflict between groups. Importantly, such emotions can facilitate bonding between groups in the absence of group-level conflict, as is the case in bonobos as well as humans (Moscovice et al. 2019; Cheng et al. 2022). Jung referred to such forms of sociality as 'the orderly cohesion of the tribe' and 'the welfare and development of the tribe' facilitated by exogamous affiliation between groups (Jung 1983: 69–70 and 66).

The Evolution of Adolescence and the Default Mode Network: From Primary to Secondary Consciousness

In the previous discussion I have argued that the development of human consciousness as we find it in modern humans would have required an extension of life history or ontogeny to include an adolescent period of growth and that this may have occurred with *Homo erectus* during the middle Pleistocene as 'life histories near those of living humans would be expected to arise as [hominin] brain size crested 1000 cc' (Smith and Tompkins 1995: 264). Of course, we cannot be certain about these things – however, it is unlikely that an adolescent period of growth, with the associated heterochronic shifts in the ontogeny of brain development, existed in small-brained hominins such as *Ardipithecus ramidus* and the Australopithecines. The process of heterochronic alteration of ontogeny from a primate-like life history to a human one is consequently most likely no older than 2 million years – although it is possible it occurred more recently.

In primates, and particularly in humans, there are important heterochronic shifts in brain maturation with the extension of the period of development of cortical regions – as was noted above in the discussion of human brain ontogeny. The result of such alterations in the timing of brain maturation means that cortical neurogenesis is protracted, whereas limbic neurogenesis is shortened (Charvet, Striedter, and Finlay 2011). In humans, this means that the deeper parts of the brain develop during embryogenesis, with cortical regions maturing much later in development (Finlay and Darlington 1995).

Importantly, such heterochronic shifts in brain ontogeny may translate into synaptic activity and metabolism differences between adult humans and chimpanzees, resulting in the enhancement of learning and cultural transmission in humans (Somel, Rohlfs, and Liu 2014). In such shifts, we can see how Haeckel's notion of heterochrony is applied in modern evolutionary brain research and how the extension of ontogenetic growth trajectories in humans may be an important factor that distinguishes our unique form of psychology from other primates. Summarising this ontogenetic trajectory of brain maturation, Jones writes that the 'higher-order association cortices mature after lower-order somatosensory and visual cortices' and that 'phylogenetically older brain areas mature earlier than those more recently evolved such as the frontal cortex' (Jones 2013: 9). Jung made a similar point when he wrote that 'consciousness is phylogenetically and ontogenetically a secondary phenomenon' (Jung 2011: 348).

Alan Hobson has developed an approach that in a very similar manner to Jung, proposes a parallel between ontogeny and phylogeny. For Hobson, the ontogenetic transition from primary to secondary consciousness reflects a similar transition in phylogeny. This approach is based on the assumption that primary consciousness precedes secondary consciousness both in individual development and in the evolution of our species. As he writes:

> The proto-consciousness and the psychoanalytic model probably share the conviction that primary consciousness (or process) is more ontogenetically and phylogenetically primitive than secondary consciousness (or process). Newborn infants and lower animals possess primary conscious states in full measure. An important point is that these relatively primitive primary states are brain-mind functions that depend upon the lower brain while the secondary states only develop when the cortico-thalamic system of the upper brain matures (especially in the developing human). While most animals, young and old, human and subhuman, have subcortical brains of comparable complexity, the complexity of the upper brain increases markedly in the early development of each lifetime and over eons of evolutionary time in the origin of the species.
>
> (Hobson 2014: 109)

This secondary process or higher order network in humans comprises a centrally situated hub of brain activity that links parts of the cerebral cortex to deeper, older structures in the brain, such as the limbic system and the hippocampus. As already noted, this central control hub has been termed the default mode network by neuroscientists (Raichle et al. 2001; Raichle and Snyder 2007). The default mode network is believed to be involved in a number of uniquely human cognitive capacities such as language and conceptual processing (Rilling et al. 2007), the construction of autobiographical narratives, the ability to project the self into the future, theory of mind as well as the uniquely human sense of self or ego (Rilling et al. 2007; Raichle and Snyder 2007; Spreng, Mar, and Kim 2008; Spreng and Grady 2010; Carhart-Harris and Friston 2010). Significantly, the default mode network is believed to be the basis of secondary consciousness and the self-reflective capacities of the human ego complex studied by Freud and Jung (Carhart-Harris and Friston 2010; Carhart-Harris et al. 2014). As mentioned above this network may have been recruited in *Homo erectus* tool manufacture (Stout et al. 2015).

In humans, the default mode network goes through a number of changes throughout ontogeny and its full maturation seems to be related to our extended life history pattern. Importantly, human infants do not possess a default mode network like that of adults. This is thought to be the related to the lack of adult-like self-referential processing and mental projection in time in infant cognition (Fransson et al. 2007). In adults the default mode network is thought to be related to the structural and functional integration between the medial prefrontal cortex and the posterior cingulate cortex. It has been found that children between seven and nine years of age lack the adult degree of interconnectivity between these two regions of the brain (Fair et al. 2008). Research comparing children with young adults has indicated increased functional integration between the medial prefrontal cortex and the posterior cingulate cortex occurs to during adolescence. It is at this developmental stage that adult like social cognition and intellectual capabilities begin to develop (Supekar et al. 2010). The essential point is that infants and children have a default mode network unlike the configuration evident in adolescents and adults. Importantly, it is during the adolescent period that we see not only maturation of the default mode network but also a transition from primary to secondary consciousness – that is, from subcortical to more cortical control of behaviour (Fair et al. 2008; Jones 2013).

Importantly for clinical and therapeutic perspectives, this network has been implicated in our species unique vulnerability for developing various forms of psychopathology (Shim et al. 2010; Whitfield-Gabrieli and Ford 2012). This vulnerability seems to result from the evolution of the default mode network and secondary consciousness out of a more archaic primary process system of socio-affective consciousness (Carhart-Harris and Friston 2010; Carhart-Harris et al. 2014; Clark 2017). Significantly, Jung believed that consciousness can become 'disturbed' when it deviates from its 'archetypal, instinctual foundation' (Jung 2014a: 39–40), while Neumann argued the adolescent period of development, particularly in males, results in a vulnerability for developing hebephrenia, a form of schizophrenia typically appearing during this period in ontogeny (Neumann 1994: 250).

Jones has argued that mental illness in humans is best understood from a developmental perspective and that biological changes the brain undergoes as it transitions from childhood, through adolescence and into adulthood, underpin the vulnerability for developing psychopathology. Such maturational processes are characterised by 'a temporary uncoupling of higher-order, more recently evolved cortical functions from the limbic and subcortical systems that mature earlier.' As he elaborates:

> A 'neural maturation gap' during adolescence exists between earlier maturation of limbic and subcortical reward processing networks … and later consolidation of neocortical cognitive and emotional control networks dependent on environmental experience. This maturation gap may present a window of vulnerability during which these two different systems are not yet fully coordinated.
>
> (Jones 2013: 9)

What the above discussion suggests is that the vulnerability for developing psychopathology that characterises our species, is a result of the evolution of our unique cognitive ontogeny. In this sense it is unlikely that early hominins such as *Ardipithecus ramidus* developed forms of psychopathology of the kind that characterises more recent periods of hominin evolution. While there are still many uncertainties at play here, I suspect that such vulnerabilities are related to the extension of our life history to include childhood and adolescent periods of somatic and brain development. In this sense, they probably emerged in *Homo erectus* when we begin to see a modern human-like pattern of brain development. We may speculate that with this group of hominins ritual technologies for altering the interactions between different brain systems may have first developed, giving at least some credence to the controversial 'stoned ape' theory of human evolution (McKenna 1999). Importantly, sociocultural factors are important in the aetiology of modern forms of psychopathology – and these uniquely modern factors would not have characterised *Homo erectus* social life.

There is also very suggestive evidence that as brain size increases, segregation between different brain regions also increases. This is because as brain size increases, brain regions move further apart from one another, which makes interactions between such regions more difficult; as Striedter writes an 'ancestral brain region' may become 'subdivided, or "segregated," into two or more brain regions in a descendant' (Striedter 2004: 180). Such segregation may be important for normal brain function and behaviour. As Striedter elaborates as 'complexity increases,' brain areas 'specialize for different functions, leading to improved performance on at least some tasks.' As a result of this process 'brain regions tend to fractionate into more subdivisions, nuclei, or areas as they enlarge phylogenetically' (Striedter 2004: 10). As Striedter elaborates:

> … connection density (the proportion of a brain's neurons that are interconnected directly) tends to decrease as neuron number increases. This rule arises naturally from the fact that individual neurons are limited in how many other neurons they can innervate (or receive input from); it is functionally significant because without it, neuronal wiring costs would increase exponentially with increasing brain size. Decreasing connection density also forces brains to become

more modular, by which I mean that distant brain regions become functionally more independent and diverse. Up to a point, this increased modularity is beneficial but too much modularity impedes coordination.

(Striedter 2004: 11)

One of the possible results of this process is that as regions become disproportionately large, 'they tend to "invade" regions that they did not innervate ancestrally' which may result in the enlarged, invading region becoming 'more important for normal brain function and behavior' (Striedter 2004: 11). It is hard to know if such conceptions of brain evolution, which are derived from living species, can be legitimately applied to fossil hominins. However, it is not inconceivable that as brain size increased not only was ontogeny extended but that brain regions also became more segregated. It is interesting to speculate that such segregation may underpin the dissociation Jung referred to when he argued that consciousness can become 'disturbed' deviating from its 'archetypal, instinctual foundation' creating a relationship of opposition between consciousness and the unconscious. (Jung 2014a: 39–40). If this view has any validity, then it implies that the human brain is biologically predisposed to become segregated or dissociated – or as Jung would describe it opposition between consciousness and the unconscious. Such an approach would explain why altered states and ritualistic forms of healing seem to involve both a regression to more ancient brain systems and desegregation of neural architecture – an issue I take up in more detail in the next chapter.

Jonathan Burns, in his *The Descent of Madness: Evolutionary Origins of Psychosis and the Social Brain*, develops a similar approach to that outlined above. As he writes, 'psychosis, and schizophrenia in particular, should be considered a costly by-product of social brain evolution in *Homo sapiens*' and that 'the evolution of complex cortical circuits' is the 'key to both modern human social cognition and behaviour, and our species' capacity for psychotic illness.' As he elaborates:

Any discussion of cerebral connectivity must include a review of the mechanisms involved in the development and maturation of the brain itself. Specifically, any evolutionary discourse on cerebral connectivity must include an analysis of how neurodevelopmental processes have changed during evolution. Such discussion and analysis will … allow us to speculate about abnormal developmental processes in the genesis of the schizophrenic brain.

(Burns 2007)

The evolutionary changes to neurodevelopmental processes Burns is referring to is essentially the alteration of ontogeny or life history during hominin phylogenesis I have discussed above.

Alison Gopnik and colleagues have explored the ontogeny of such changes and the process of brain maturation we undergo as we age. Intriguingly they found that very young children outperform adults on a number of cognitive tasks, suggesting, somewhat counter-intuitively, that as we age certain aspects of cognitive performance decrease. This seems to be associated with development of the pre-frontal cortex during which neural plasticity as well as divergent and exploratory thinking decline. This decline of exploratory and divergent thinking however is re-placed by a more secure and informed knowledge of the world. As Gopnik and col-leagues write, adult cognition excels at 'the tried and true, while children are more likely to discover the weird and wonderful. This may be because as we get older, we both know more and explore less' (Gopnik, Griffiths, and Lucas 2015: 91).

This developmental transformation seems to be associated with the prolifera-tion of synaptic connections during the early stages of ontogeny, with a subse-quent stage of synaptic pruning occurring as we mature. The consequence of these changes is that the brain is transformed from a state of flexibility and sensitivity into a more 'effective and controlled' state (Gopnik et al. 2017: 7893). Signifi-cantly, the transition from childhood cognitive styles to those of adulthood involve a reduction in entropy and increased order and rigidity as secondary consciousness and the default mode network mature (Carhart-Harris et al. 2014; Carhart-Harris and Friston 2019).

In Gopnik's view, adults can recapture the more flexible, exploratory, less or-dered and entropic brain state characteristic of the early stages of ontogeny. It is this ability that underpins human creativity which involves 'disruptions to fron-tal control' resulting 'in a more "child-like" brain' with improved performance in cognitive tasks that involve exploring a wide range of possibilities (Gopnik et al. 2015: 91). Elaborating on this line of thinking Gopnik notes that certain environ-ments 'may lead to more flexible, exploratory and childlike learning, even in adult-hood' (Gopnik et al. 2017: 7898). Significantly, Gopnik uses these findings in a broader analysis of culture that is pertinent to the themes of this study:

> Scientists have other words for mess: variability, stochasticity, noise, entropy, randomness. A long tradition, going back to the Greek rationalist philosophers, sees these forces of disorder as the enemies of knowledge, progress, and civili-zation. But another tradition, going back to the nineteenth-century Romantics, sees disorder as the wellspring of freedom, innovation, and creativity. The Ro-mantics also celebrated childhood; for them, children were the quintessential example of the virtues of chaos. New science provides some ammunition for the Romantic view. From brains to babies to robots to scientists, mess has merits. A system that shifts and varies, even randomly, can adapt to a changing world in a more intelligent and flexible way.
>
> (Gopnik 2016: 26)

Alan Hobson has proposed a similar approach; for example, the cognitive style characteristic of childhood seems to have greater affinity with dream mentation and creativity than that of adult cognitive styles. As he writes:

> Thus the brain of one and all is fundamentally artistic. We know this when we see the drawings of our children, but tend to discount it in our adult lives.

So highly socialised are we to accept our given wake-state role that we fail to recognise the clear-cut evidence of our dreams that each of us possesses creative ability. Each of us is a surrealist at night during his or her dreams: each is a Picasso, a Dali, a Fellini – the delightful and the macabre mixed in full measure.

(Hobson 1989: 297)

The above discussion offers possible evolutionary developmental perspectives on Jung's archetype of the child and rebirth motif and their importance for the process of individuation. As Jung writes this archetype represents a 'maturation process of personality' during which 'preconscious processes, gradually pass over into the conscious mind, or become conscious as dreams' (Jung 2014a: 159).

Elsewhere I explored the child and rebirth archetypes in a neurophenomenological analysis of *Faust* (Clark 2022). Goethe's theory of art and his development of the rebirth motif are evident in the transformation of Faust into a boy at the end of the play and his admittance into the choir of blessed youths. However, as I argued, such examples of the child archetype and a phase transition to the early periods of ontogeny do not represent a nostalgic regression from adulthood to earlier stages of development, but the' incorporation and freshness of childhood perception into the higher maturity of adulthood' (Abrams 1971: 380; Clark 2022: 320). It is likely that such a state of freshness, evident in the work of Goethe and central to Jung's concept of the child archetype, is instantiated when neural hierarchies associated with our extended life history and cognitive ontogeny are obviated.

References

Abrams, M.H. 1971. *Natural Supernaturalism: Tradition and Revolution in Romantic Literature* (Norton).

Antón, S.C., and S.R. Leigh. 2003. 'Growth and Life History in Homo erectus.' in Krovitz, G.E., A.J. Nelson and J.L. Thompson (eds.), *Patterns of Growth and Development in the Genus Homo* (Cambridge University Press).

Arsuaga, J.L. 2009. *The Neanderthal's Necklace: In Search of the First Thinkers* (Basic Books).

Bachofen, J.J. 1967. *Myth, Religion, and Mother Right: Selected Writings of J. J. Bachofen* (Routledge).

Bednarik, R.G. 2015. *The First Mariners* (Bentham Science Publishers).

Benítez-Burraco, A., and V. Kempe. 2018. 'The Emergence of Modern Languages: Has Human Self-Domestication Optimized Language Transmission?', *Frontiers in Psychology*, 9: 1–8.

Bogin, B. 2003. 'The Human Pattern of Growth and Development in Paleontological Perspective.' in Nelson, A.J., G.E. Krovitz and J.L. Thompson (eds.), *Patterns of Growth and Development in the Genus Homo* (Cambridge University Press).

Bogin, B., and B. H. Smith. 1996. 'Evolution of the Human Life Cycle', *American Journal of Human Biology*, 8: 703–16.

Boyer, P. 2008. *Religion Explained* (Random House).

Boesch, C. 2009. *The Real Chimpanzee: Sex Strategies in the Forest* (Cambridge University Press).

Brooks, J., F. Kano, Y. Kawaguchi, S. Yamamoto. 2022. 'Oxytocin Promotes Species-Relevant Outgroup Attention in Bonobos and Chimpanzees', *Hormones and Behavior*, 143: 1–11.

Brunet, M., F. Guy, D. Pilbeam, H.T. Mackaye, A. Likius, D. Ahounta, et al. 2002. 'A New Hominid from the Upper Miocene of Chad, Central Africa', *Nature*, 418: 145–51.

Burns, J. 2007. *The Descent of Madness: Evolutionary Origins of Psychosis and the Social Brain* (Taylor & Francis).

Carhart-Harris, R.L., and K.J. Friston. 2010. 'The Default-Mode, Ego-Functions and Free-Energy: A Neurobiological Account of Freudian Ideas', *Brain*, 133: 1265–83.

Carhart-Harris, R.L., and K.J. Friston. 2019. 'REBUS and the Anarchic Brain: Toward a Unified Model of the Brain Action of Psychedelics', *Pharmacological Reviews*, 71: 316.

Carhart-Harris, R.L., R. Leech, P.J. Hellyer, M. Shanahan, A. Feilding, E. Tagliazucchi, et al. 2014. 'The Entropic Brain: A Theory of Conscious States Informed by Neuroimaging Research with Psychedelic Drugs', *Frontiers in Human Neuroscience*, 8: 1–22.

Cela-Conde, C.J., and F.J. Ayala. 2007. *Human Evolution: Trails from the Past* (OUP Oxford).

Charvet, C.J., G.F. Striedter, and B.L. Finlay. 2011. 'Evo-Devo and Brain Scaling: Candidate Developmental Mechanisms for Variation and Constancy in Vertebrate Brain Evolution', *Brain Behavior and Evolution*, 78: 248–57.

Chen, S., and W. Chen. 2016. 'A Chain of Tools: An Experimental Study on Picks of the Qinling Region', *Quaternary International*, 400: 93–9.

Cheng, L., L. Samuni, S. Lucchesi, T. Deschner, and M. Surbeck. 2022. 'Love thy neighbour: Behavioural and Endocrine Correlates of Male Strategies during Intergroup Encounters in Bonobos', *Animal Behaviour*, 187: 319–30.

Churchland, P.S. 2018. *Braintrust: What Neuroscience Tells Us about Morality* (Princeton University Press).

Clark, G. 2017. 'The Dionysian Primate: The Default Mode Network, Psychopathology and the Psychedelic Brain.' In *Entheogenesis Australis Psychedelic Symposium 2017*, 25–27. Victoria Australia: Entheogenesis Australis.

Clark, G. 2022. 'The Dionysian Primate: Goethe, Nietzsche, Jung and Psychedelic Neuroscience.' in Miils, J., and D. Burston (eds.), *Psychoanalysis and the Mind-Body Problem* (Routledge).

Clark, G., and M. Henneberg. 2017. 'Ardipithecus ramidus and the Evolution of Language and Singing: An Early Origin for Hominin Vocal Capability', *HOMO – Journal of Comparative Human Biology*, 68: 101–21.

Clark, G., and M. Henneberg. 2021a. 'Cognitive and Behavioral Modernity in Homo erectus: Skull Globularity and Hominin Brain Evolution', *Anthropological Review*, 84: 467–85.

Clark, G., and M. Henneberg. 2021b. 'Interpopulational Variation in Human Brain Size: Implications for Hominin Cognitive Phylogeny', *Anthropological Review*, 84: 405–29.

Clark, Gary, and Maciej Henneberg. 2015. 'The Life History of Ardipithecus ramidus: A Heterochronic Model of Sexual and Social Maturation', *Anthropological Review*, 78: 109–32.

Corballis, M.C. 2019. Language, Memory, and Mental Time Travel: An Evolutionary Perspective. *Frontiers in Human Neuroscience*, 13: 1–9.

Dean, C., M.G. Leakey, D. Reid, F. Schrenk, G.T. Schwartz, C. Stringer, et al. 2001. 'Growth Processes in Teeth Distinguish Modern Humans from Homo erectus and Earlier Hominins', *Nature*, 414: 628–31.

Dean, M.C., and H.M. Liversidge. 2015. 'Age Estimation in Fossil Hominins: Comparing Dental Development in Early Homo with Modern Humans', *Annals of Human Biology*, 42: 415–29.

Dean, M.C., and B.H. Smith. 2009. 'Growth and Development of the Nariokotome Youth, KNM-WT 15000.' in Fleagle, J.G., F.E. Grine and R.E. Leakey (eds.), *The First Humans – Origin and Early Evolution of the Genus Homo* (Springer).

Diamond, J.M. 2006. *The Third Chimpanzee: The Evolution and Future of the Human Animal* (HarperCollins).

Dissanayake, E. 2021. 'Ancestral Human Mother-Infant Interaction Was an Adaptation that Gave Rise to Music and Dance', *Behavioral and Brain Sciences*, 44: e68.

Dugatkin, L. 2007. 'Inclusive Fitness Theory from Darwin to Hamilton', *Genetics*, 176: 1375–80.

Dunbar, R. 2014. *Human Evolution: A Pelican Introduction* (Penguin Books Limited).

Dunbar, R. 2022. *How Religion Evolved: And Why It Endures* (Oxford University Press).

Durkheim, É. 2008. *The Elementary Forms of Religious Life* (OUP Oxford).

Fair, D.A., A.L. Cohen, N.U.F. Dosenbach, J.A. Church, F.M. Miezin, D.M. Barch, et al. 2008. 'The Maturing Architecture of the Brain's Default Network', *Proceedings of the National Academy of Sciences*, 105: 4028–32.

Falk, D. 2016. 'Evolution of Brain and Culture: The Neurological and Cognitive Journey from Australopithecus to Albert Einstein', *Journal of Anthropological Sciences*, 94: 99–111.

Finlay, B.L., and R.B. Darlington. 1995. 'Linked Regularities in the Development and Evolution of Mammalian Brains', *Science*, 268: 1578–84.

Fransson, P., B. Skiold, S. Horsch, A. Nordell, M. Blennow, H. Lagercrantz, et al. 2007. 'Resting-State Networks in the Infant Brain', *Proceedings of the National Academy of Sciences*, 104: 15531–6.

Furuichi, T., and J. Thompson. 2007. *The Bonobos: Behavior, Ecology, and Conservation* (Springer New York).

Geary, D.C., and M. Flinn. 2001. 'Evolution of Human Parental Behavior and the Human Family', *Parenting*, 1: 5–61.

Gopnik, A. 2016. *The Gardener and the Carpenter: What the New Science of Child Development Tells Us about the Relationship between Parents and Children* (Farrar, Straus and Giroux).

Gopnik, A., T.L. Griffiths, and C.G. Lucas. 2015. 'When Younger Learners Can Be Better (or at Least More Open-Minded) than Older Ones', *Current Directions in Psychological Science*, 24: 87–92.

Gopnik, A., S. O'Grady, C.G. Lucas, T.L. Griffiths, A. Wente, S. Bridgers, et al. 2017. 'Changes in Cognitive Flexibility and Hypothesis Search across Human Life History from Childhood to Adolescence to Adulthood', *Proceedings of the National Academy of Sciences*, 114: 7892–9.

Gordon, A. 2013. 'Sexual Size Dimorphism in Australopithecus: Current Understanding and New Directions.' in Kaye, E.R., John G.F., and Richard E.L. (eds.), *The Paleobiology of Australopithecus* (Springer Netherlands).

Gordon, I., O. Zagoory-Sharon, J.F. Leckman, and R. Feldman. 2010. 'Prolactin, Oxytocin, and the Development of Paternal Behavior across the First Six Months of Fatherhood', *Hormones and Behavior*, 58: 513–8.

Harvey, A.R. 2020. 'Links Between the Neurobiology of Oxytocin and Human Musicality', *Frontiers in Human Neuroscience*, 14: 1–19.

Haile-Selassie, Y., G. Suwa, and T.D. White. 2004. 'Late Miocene Teeth from Middle Awash, Ethiopia, and Early Hominid Dental Evolution', *Science*, 303: 1503–5.

Haile-Selassie, Y., and G. WoldeGabriel. 2009. *Ardipithecus Kadabba: Late Miocene Evidence from the Middle Awash, Ethiopia* (University of California Press).

Hall, B.K. 1993. *Evolutionary Developmental Biology* (Springer Netherlands).

Hall, B.K. 2011. 'Ontogeny does not recapitulate phylogeny, it creates phylogeny: a review of The Tragic Sense of Life: Ernst Haeckel and the Struggle over Evolutionary Thought, by Robert J. Richards.' Wiley Online Library.

Hamilton, W.D. 1964a. 'The Genetical Evolution of Social Behaviour. I', *Journal of Theoretical Biology*, 7: 1–16.

Hamilton, W.D. 1964b. 'The Genetical Evolution of Social Behaviour. II', *Journal of Theoretical Biology*, 7: 17–52.

Hare, B. 2017. 'Survival of the Friendliest: Homo sapiens Evolved via Selection for Prosociality', *Annual Review of Psychology*, 68: 155–86.

Hashimoto, C., Y. Tashiro, E. Hibino, M. Mulavwa, K. Yangozene, T. Furuichi, et al. 2008. 'Longitudinal Structure of a Unit-Group of Bonobos: Male Philopatry and Possible Fusion of Unit-Groups.' in Furuichi, T., and J. Thompson (eds.), *The Bonobos: Behavior, Ecology, and Conservation* (Springer New York).

Hawkes, K., and R.R. Paine. 2006. *The Evolution of Human Life History* (School of American Research).

Herries, A.I.R., J.M. Martin, A.B. Leece, J.W. Adams, G. Boschian, R. Joannes-Boyau, et al. 2020. 'Contemporaneity of Australopithecus, Paranthropus, and Early Homo erectus in South Africa', *Science*, 368: eaaw7293.

Hobson, A. 1989. *The Dreaming Brain* (Basic Books).

Hobson, A. 2014. *Psychodynamic Neurology: Dreams, Consciousness, and Virtual Reality* (Taylor & Francis).

Hoffmann, D., D. Angelucci, V. Villaverde, J. Zapata, and J. Zilhão. 2018. 'Symbolic Use of Marine Shells and Mineral Pigments by Iberian Neandertals 115,000 Years Ago', *Science Advances*, 4: eaar5255.

Hublin, J.J., S. Neubauer, and P. Gunz. 2015. 'Brain Ontogeny and Life History in Pleistocene Hominins', *Philosophical Transactions of the Royal Society of London B: Biological Sciences*, 370: 20140062.

Itani, G. 1990. 'Relations between Unit-Groups of Bonobos at Wamba, Zaire: Encounters and Temporary Fusions', *African Study Monographs*, 11: 153–86.

Jaubert, J., S. Verheyden, D. Genty, M. Soulier, H. Cheng, and D. Blamart, et al. 2016. 'Early Neanderthal Constructions Deep in Bruniquel Cave in Southwestern France', *Nature*, 534: 111–4.

Jones, P.B. 2013. 'Adult Mental Health Disorders and Their Age at Onset', *The British Journal of Psychiatry*, 202: s5–s10.

Jung, C.G. 1960. *The Collected Works of C.G. Jung: The Psychogenesis of Mental Disease* (Routledge & Kegan Paul).

Jung, C.G. 1970. *Mysterium Coniunctionis: An Inquiry into the Separation and Synthesis of Psychic Opposites in Alchemy* (Princeton University Press).

Jung, C.G. 1983. *The Psychology of the Transference* (Routledge).

Jung, C.G. 1998. *Visions: Notes of the Seminar Given in 1930-1934* (Routledge).

Jung, C.G. 2011. *Memories, Dreams, Reflections* (Knopf Doubleday Publishing Group).

Jung, C.G. 2014a. *Collected Works of C.G. Jung, Volume 9 (Part 1): Archetypes and the Collective Unconscious* (Princeton University Press).

Jung, C.G. 2014b. *Collected Works of C.G. Jung, Volume 18: The Symbolic Life: Miscellaneous Writings* (Princeton University Press).

Jung, C.G. 2014c. *The Structure and Dynamics of the Psyche* (Taylor & Francis).

Jung, C.G. 2014d. *Symbols of Transformation* (Taylor & Francis).

Jung, C.G. 2020. *C.G. Jung Speaking: Interviews and Encounters* (Princeton University Press).

Laland, K., C. Wilkins, and N. Clayton. 2016. 'The Evolution of Dance', *Current Biology*, 26: R5–R9.

Lathouwers, M., and L. Elsacker. 2005. 'Reproductive Parameters of FemalePan Paniscus and P. troglodytes: Quality versus Quantity', *International Journal of Primatology*, 26: 55–71.

Light, K.C., K.M. Grewen, and J.A. Amico. 2005. 'More Frequent Partner Hugs and Higher Oxytocin Levels Are Linked to Lower Blood Pressure and Heart Rate in Premenopausal Women', *Biological Psychology*, 69: 5–21.

Locke, J., and B. Bogin. 2006. 'Language and Life History: A New Perspective on the Development and Evolution of Human Language', *Behavioral and Brain Sciences*, 29: 259–325.

Lovejoy, C.O. 2009. 'Reexamining Human Origins in Light of Ardipithecus ramidus', *Science*, 326: 74–74, 74e1–74e8.

Lovejoy, O., B. Latimer, G. Suwa, B. Asfaw, and T. White. 2009. 'Combining Prehension and Propulsion: The Foot of Ardipithecus ramidus', *Science*, 326: 72–72e8.

Mayr, E. 1963. 'The Taxonomic Evaluation of Fossil Hominids.' in Washburn, S.L. (ed.), *Classification and Human Evolution* (Routledge).

McKenna, T. 1999. *Food of the Gods: The Search for the Original Tree of Knowledge: A Radical History of Plants, Drugs and Human Evolution* (Rider).

Minugh-Purvis, N., and K.J. McNamara. 2002. *Human Evolution through Developmental Change* (Johns Hopkins University Press).

Moscovice, L., M. Surbeck, B. Fruth, G. Hohmann, A. Jaeggi, and T. Deschner. 2019. 'The Cooperative Sex: Sexual Interactions among Female Bonobos Are Linked to Increases in Oxytocin, Proximity and Coalitions', *Hormones and Behavior*, 116: 104581.

Neumann, E. 1994. *The Fear of the Feminine: And Other Essays on Feminine Psychology* (Princeton University Press).

Okasha, S. 2006. *Evolution and the Levels of Selection* (Clarendon Press).

Otis, L. 1994. *Organic Memory: History and the Body in the Late Nineteenth & Early Twentieth Centuries* (University of Nebraska Press).

Pääbo, S. 2014. *Neanderthal Man: In Search of Lost Genomes* (Basic Books).

Panksepp, J. 2004. *Affective Neuroscience: The Foundations of Human and Animal Emotions* (Oxford University Press).

Panksepp, J., and L. Biven. 2012. *The Archaeology of Mind: Neuroevolutionary Origins of Human Emotions* (W. W. Norton).

Preston, S. D. 2013. 'The Origins of Altruism in Offspring Care', *Psychological Bulletin*, 139: 1305.

Preston, S.D. 2022. *The Altruistic Urge: Why We're Driven to Help Others* (Columbia University Press).

Prüfer, K., F. Racimo, N. Patterson, F. Jay, S. Sankararaman, and S. Sawyer. 2014. 'The Complete Genome Sequence of a Neanderthal from the Altai Mountains', *Nature*, 505: 43–9.

Raichle, M.E., A.M. MacLeod, A.Z. Snyder, W.J. Powers, D.A. Gusnard, and G.L. Shulman. 2001. 'A Default Mode of Brain Function', *Proceedings of the National Academy of Sciences*, 98: 676–82.

Raichle, M., and A. Snyder. 2007. 'A Default Mode of Brain Function: A Brief History of an Evolving Idea', *NeuroImage*, 37: 1083–90.

Reno, P.L., and C. Owen Lovejoy. 2015. 'From Lucy to Kadanuumuu: Balanced Analyses of Australopithecus afarensis Assemblages Confirm Only Moderate Skeletal Dimorphism', *PeerJ*, 3: e925.

Reno, P.L., R.S. Meindl, M.A. McCollum, and C. Owen Lovejoy. 2003. 'Sexual Dimorphism in Australopithecus afarensis Was Similar to that of Modern Humans', *Proceedings of the National Academy of Sciences*, 100: 9404–9.

Richards, R.J. 2000. 'Kant and Blumenbach on the Bildungstrieb: A Historical Misunderstanding', *Studies in History and Philosophy of Science Part C: Studies in History and Philosophy of Biological and Biomedical Sciences*, 31: 11–32.

Rilling, J.K., S.K. Barks, L.A. Parr, T.M. Preuss, T.L. Faber, G. Pagnoni, et al. 2007. 'A Comparison of Resting-State Brain Activity in Humans and Chimpanzees', *Proceedings of the National Academy of Sciences*, 104: 17146–51.

Rilling, J.K., A.C. DeMarco, P.D. Hackett, R. Thompson, B. Ditzen, R. Patel, et al. 2012. 'Effects of Intranasal Oxytocin and Vasopressin on Cooperative Behavior and Associated Brain Activity in Men', *Psychoneuroendocrinology*, 37: 447–61.

Roebroeks, W., M.J. Sier, T.K. Nielsen, D. De Loecker, J.M. Parés, C.E.S. Arps, et al. 2012. 'Use of Red Ochre by Early Neandertals', *Proceedings of the National Academy of Sciences*, 109: 1889–94.

Samuni, L., A. Preis, R. Mundry, T. Deschner, C. Crockford, and R.M. Wittig. 2017. 'Oxytocin Reactivity during Intergroup Conflict in Wild Chimpanzees', *Proceedings of the National Academy of Sciences of the United States of America*, 114: 268–73.

Sayers, K., M.A. Raghanti, and C.O. Lovejoy. 2012. 'Human Evolution and the Chimpanzee Referential Doctrine', *Annual Review of Anthropology*, 41: 119–38.

Shim, G., J.S. Oh, W. Jung, J. Jang, C.-H. Choi, E. Kim, et al. 2010. 'Altered Resting-State Connectivity in Subjects at Ultra-High Risk for Psychosis: An fMRI Study', *Behavioral and Brain Functions*, 6: 58.

Smith, B.H., and R.L. Tompkins. 1995. 'Toward a Life History of the Hominidae', *Annual Review of Anthropology*, 24: 257–79.

Somel, M., R. Rohlfs, and X. Liu. 2014. 'Transcriptomic Insights into Human Brain Evolution: Acceleration, Neutrality, Heterochrony', *Current Opinion in Genetics & Development*, 29: 110–9.

Spreng, R.N., and C.L. Grady. 2010. 'Patterns of Brain Activity Supporting Autobiographical Memory, Prospection, and Theory of Mind, and Their Relationship to the Default Mode Network', *Journal of Cognitive Neuroscience*, 22: 1112–23.

Spreng, R.N., R.A. Mar, and A.S.N. Kim. 2008. 'The Common Neural Basis of Autobiographical Memory, Prospection, Navigation, Theory of Mind, and the Default Mode: A Quantitative Meta-Analysis', *Journal of Cognitive Neuroscience*, 21: 489–510.

Sterelny, K. 2012. *The Evolved Apprentice* (MIT Press).

Stout, D., E. Hecht, N. Khreisheh, B. Bradley, and T. Chaminade. 2015. 'Cognitive Demands of Lower Paleolithic Toolmaking', *PLOS ONE*, 10: e0121804.

Striedter, G.F. 2004. *Brain Evolution* (Sinauer).

Supekar, K., L.Q. Uddin, K. Prater, H. Amin, M.D. Greicius, and V. Menon. 2010. 'Development of Functional and Structural Connectivity within the Default Mode Network in Young Children', *NeuroImage*, 52: 290–301.

Suwa, G., B. Asfaw, R.T. Kono, D. Kubo, C.O. Lovejoy, and T.D. White. 2009. 'The Ardipithecus ramidus Skull and Its Implications for Hominid Origins', *Science*, 326: 68, 68e1–68e7.

Suwa, G., T. Sasaki, S. Semaw, M.J. Rogers, S.W. Simpson, Y. Kunimatsu, et al. 2021. 'Canine Sexual Dimorphism in Ardipithecus ramidus Was Nearly Human-Like', *Proceedings of the National Academy of Sciences of the United States of America*, 118: 1–11.

Trevathan, W., and K.R. Rosenberg. 2016. *Costly and Cute: Helpless Infants and Human Evolution* (University of New Mexico Press).

Turk, M., I. Turk, L. Dimkaroski, B.A.B. Blackwell, F.Z. Horusitzky, M. Otte, et al. 2018. 'The Mousterian Musical Instrument from the Divje Babe I Cave (Slovenia): Arguments on the Material Evidence for Neanderthal Musical Behaviour', *L'anthropologie*, 122: 679–706.

Walker, A., and P. Shipman. 2005. *The Ape in the Tree: An Intellectual & Natural History of Proconsul* (Belknap Press of Harvard University Press).

White, T.D., C.O. Lovejoy, B. Asfaw, J.P. Carlson, and G. Suwa. 2015. 'Neither Chimpanzee nor Human, Ardipithecus Reveals the Surprising Ancestry of Both', *Proceedings of the National Academy of Sciences of the United States of America*, 112: 4877–84.

White, T.D., G. Suwa, and C.O. Lovejoy. 2010. 'Response to Comment on the Paleobiology and Classification of *Ardipithecus ramidus*', *Science*, 328: 1105.

Whitfield-Gabrieli, S., and J.M. Ford. 2012. 'Default Mode Network Activity and Connectivity in Psychopathology', *Annual Review of Clinical Psychology*, 8: 49–76.

Wilson, D. 2003. *Darwin's Cathedral: Evolution, Religion, and the Nature of Society* (University of Chicago Press).

Wilson, D.S., and E.O. Wilson. 2007. 'Rethinking the Theoretical Foundation of Sociobiology', *The Quarterly Review of Biology*, 82: 327–48.

Wilson, E.O. 2012. *The Social Conquest of Earth* (Liveright).

Wynn, T. 1989. *The Evolution of Spatial Competence* (University of Illinois Press).

Xing, S., P. Tafforeau, M. O'Hara, M. Modesto-Mata, L. Martín-Francés, M. Martinón-Torres, et al. 2019. 'First Systematic Assessment of Dental Growth and Development in an Archaic Hominin (genus, Homo) from East Asia', *Science Advances*, 5: eaau0930.

Zhou, C., Z. Liu, Y. Wang, and Q. Huang. 2000. 'Climatic Cycles Investigated by Sediment Analysis in Peking Man's Cave, Zhoukoudian, China', *Journal of Archaeological Science*, 27: 101–9.

Zilhão, J., D.E. Angelucci, E. Badal-García, F. d'Errico, F. Daniel, L. Dayet, et al. 2010. 'Symbolic Use of Marine Shells and Mineral Pigments by Iberian Neandertals', *Proceedings of the National Academy of Sciences*, 107: 1023–8.

Chapter 5

Analytical Psychology and the Adaptationist Paradigm

Jung and Altered States of Consciousness

Introduction

This chapter explores altered states of consciousness, psychedelic neuroscience and archaeological evidence that Palaeolithic cave art may represent depictions of trance states. The evidence surveyed suggests that trance states and the human proclivity to alter consciousness cannot be exhaustively explained as evolutionary adaptations, but most likely represent, as Jung suggested, cultural practices designed to integrate archaic and recently evolved brain systems.

Jung, Altered States of Consciousness and the Adaptationist Paradigm

In his *Big Dreams: The Science of Dreaming and the Origins of Religion*, Kelly Bulkeley presents cognitive science data that he argues supports the theories of Edward Tylor (1832–1917), Frederick Netizsche (1844–1900) and Jung regarding the association between dreamlife and the origins of religion and belief in spirits. For example, in *Human, All Too Human*, Nietzsche wrote:

> In ages of crude, primordial cultures, man thought he could come to know a second real world in dreams: this is the origin of all metaphysics. Without dreams man would have found no occasion to divide the world. The separation into body and soul is also connected to the oldest views about dreams, as is the assumption of a spiritual apparition, that is, the origin of all belief in ghosts, and probably also in gods. "The dead man lives on, because he appears to the living man in dreams." So man concluded formerly, throughout many thousands of years.
>
> (Nietzsche 1994: 16)

Jung adopted a similar approach to Tylor and Nietzsche when he wrote that '… one of the most important sources of the primitive belief in spirits is dreams. People very often appear as the actors in dreams … The dream has for him an incomparably higher value than it has for civilized man.' Jung also argued that modern Europeans do not attribute such importance to dreams of the kind we find in Indigenous and shamanic cultures. As he avers, 'if a European had to go through the same exercises and ceremonies which the medicine-man [shaman] performs in order to

DOI: 10.4324/9781032624549-6

make the spirits visible, he would have the same experiences. He would interpret them differently, of course, and devalue them' (Jung 2014b: 393).

French archaeologist and former advisor for prehistoric art at the French Ministry of Culture, Jean Clottes, has argued for a similar view to that of Jung and Nietzsche. As he writes in the foreword to David Whitley's *Cave Paintings and the Human Spirit: The Origin of Creativity and Belief* (Whitley 2009):

> I would follow in Edward Tylor's ancient footsteps and favour the emergence of spirituality from dreams – both the ordinary night dreams we all experience and the daydreams of altered states of consciousness. With the evolution of language, and the ability of people to talk about and rationalize their dreams, humans could have attributed their dream experiences to voyages to a different realm of reality, where all sorts of strange things could happen.
>
> (Clottes 2009: 20)

Clottes is addressing the issue of the possible origin of Palaeolithic cave art such as the galleries in Chauvet and Lascaux in France. Whitley develops the argument that the painting of animals in these caves may have been depictions of visionary or altered states of consciousness, which is what Clottes is alluding to. One of the pieces of evidence Whitely uses to support his argument is that the traditional explanation that the horses and bison depicted in the caves represented a form of hunting magic is not supported by the archaeological evidence. He questions this interpretation due to the simple fact that if it were correct, the animals depicted would be the same as those hunted by the inhabitants of the caves. However, as he notes, 'there is little correlation between the depicted species and excavated food remains from camp sites' (Whitley 2009: 30).

Whitely's interpretation of European Palaeolithic cave art is based on the research of South African archaeologist David Lewis-Williams. Lewis-Williams has developed at length the thesis that Palaeolithic cave art in Europe and Africa represents depictions of trance states (Lewis-Williams 2004; Lewis-Williams and Challis 2011). In *Deciphering Ancient Minds: The Mystery of San Bushman Rock Art*, Lewis-Williams made a very strong case by compiling archaeological evidence, historical documents and contemporary accounts of the San as to the meaning of the images. Summarising Lewis-Williams' conclusions on southern African rock art and ethnographic research among San foragers, Whitely writes that the 'rock surface was thought to be ... thin and permeable' representing a 'veil between the sacred and the mundane.' Contemporary San told Lewis-Williams that the images depicted on the rock surface actually represented beings that existed on the other side of the rock. During trance, shamans were believed to penetrate that surface during 'supernatural excursions.' Consequently, the paintings themselves were believed to preserve 'the images of spirits that were already within the rock and which only the shaman could see' (Whitley 2009: 39).

This seems a plausible explanation. If a shaman entered trance and sought to express or embody in communicable form, the visions that were experienced, depicting them on the rock surface, would achieve such embodiment. In this sense, inner visions could be made manifest in an external perceptible and sensory form. For Whitley, the ancient peoples of Europe similarly depicted visionary states of trance in the art at Chauvet and Lascaux – a thesis also developed at length by Lewis-Williams in his study of European Palaeolithic art, *The Mind in the Cave: Consciousness and the Origins of Art* (Lewis-Williams 2004). The converging evidence from these researchers is that early human populations used caves as places where altered and visionary states were induced – probably through ritualised dancing and music. If so, these early human cultures may have been cultivating what Jung called the *numinous* (Jung 2014b: 104).

Clottes discusses the problem of modern science, with its Enlightenment and rationalistic assumptions, investigating the art and experiential world of our Palaeolithic ancestors. This has resulted, in Clottes view, with researchers who investigate the 'evolution of cognition' emphasising 'rationality over emotion.' The consequence is that Palaeolithic art becomes potential evidence for the origins of modern cognition, for 'how reason and intellect developed, and when they first appeared.' Clottes' argues that this is an example of projecting the cultural schema of modern people's into the past; as he elaborates, 'prehistory should be understood in its own right, no explained by imposing the ways of life of recent peoples onto ancient cultures' (Clottes 2009: 15). The solution to this bias is for researchers to use Indigenous conceptions of art and religion in their reconstruction of Palaeolithic cultures, given that 'Paleolithic hunter-gatherers' ways of thinking were most likely 'closer to those of early native Americans or Australian Aborigines than to ours today' (Clottes 2009: 19). As he elaborates:

> ... to know the past requires a frame of reference that is different from our Western contemporary conception. An understanding of native American (and other traditional non-Western) cultures provides a kind of prism by which the ancient past can be examined and explored, beyond the heavy intellectual weight imposed by our Western world view. This is not a final model for how things must have worked but instead a framework that helps us overcome our contemporary – and usually unarticulated biases.
>
> (Clottes 2009: 15)

The distinction Clottes is making can be fruitfully analysed in terms of *monophasic* and *polyphasic* forms of consciousness (Laughlin, McManus, and D'Aquili 1990: 155; Laughlin 2011: 62–6). Monophasic forms of consciousness tend to be associated with cultures that disattend to dreamlife and altered states of consciousness, with an accompanying prioritisation of lucid waking rational consciousness. This is a mode of consciousness characteristic of modern Western rationalistic conceptions of mind, the attendant sense of 'ego-identification' as well as an extremely 'materialistic political economy.' Polyphasic cultural modes, which the ethnographic literature indicates are by far the most common cross-culturally, attend to dream and altered states of consciousness with the consequence that their view of the self constitutes a form of 'polyphasic integration' (Laughlin, McManus, and D'Aquili 1990: 155; Laughlin 2011: 65).

Cross-cultural analysis has found that up to 90 per cent of cultures have institutionalised means of altering consciousness. These findings have led to the conclusion that there exists a 'psychobiological capacity available to all societies' and that such utilisation occurs 'primarily in a sacred context' (Bourguignon 1973: 11). This data suggests that such experiences are an inherent aspect of our species-evolved neural architecture. Significantly, the visual phenomena experienced in such altered states are believed to arise from dissociated complexes in the unconscious that operate outside of ego consciousness – and that such a visually and emotionally rich modality represents a phylogenetically ancient form of primary consciousness based in 'somatic awareness and subjective feeling states' (Winkelman 2010: 12, 9 and 205, 2017: 7).

However, there is variation in regard to the degree to which such aspects of the brain are expressed culturally. Jung, with his wide-ranging reading in religion, ritual and anthropology, was well aware of these cultural differences. Although he did not use the term monophasic, it is essentially what he is alluding to in the above comment on dreams, and also when he avers that 'Western consciousness is by no means the only kind of consciousness there is; it is historically conditioned and geographically limited' (Jung 1953: 55). Jung's writings are essentially an attempt to incorporate polyphasic conceptions of the psyche into a modern Western scientific paradigm of consciousness.

Jung's approach however does not merely assert that altered states of consciousness are a psychobiological potentiality of our species. His approach is more nuanced and as I will argue has more explanatory power than models that see ritual and ritualised forms of dance solely as evolutionary adaptations (Wilson 2003; Dunbar 2014; Fink et al. 2021: 279–80). For example, Jung sees ritual alterations of consciousness as an attempt to integrate what may be considered antagonistic brain systems. This is an extremely important point as it suggests that cultural technologies designed to alter consciousness such as ritualised dance, music, ingestion of psychedelic compounds or meditation and yoga are not so much evolved potentialities of the brain but cultural practices designed to integrate inefficiently or inadequately integrated brain systems. Such integration presupposes an unintegrated or divided state – or what I called in Chapter 4 segregated neural architecture. Jung adopted a similar approach in his writings on the rituals of Indigenous peoples. As he writes, consciousness can become 'disturbed' deviating from its 'archetypal, instinctual foundation' creating a relationship of opposition between consciousness and the unconscious. Jung argues that Indigenous rituals such as those of Native Americans and Aboriginal Australians aim at a synthesis of these two aspects of the psyche (Jung 2014a: 39–40).

Support for Jung's more nuanced view comes from modern studies indicating reduced activity in recently evolved neural hubs such as the default mode network, as well as desegregation of brain regions, ego dissolution and a shift to right hemispheric and phylogenetically older core processes during altered states of consciousness (Flor-Henry et al. 2017; Carhart-Harris and Friston 2019; Luppi et al. 2021; Daws et al. 2022: 20). Consequently, it is crucial to start from the assumption of a segregated or disassociated brain state; otherwise, the experiential dimensions of ritual life, and their neurobiological substrates, cannot be explained. Jung seemed to be fully aware of these issues. When writing of various cross-cultural ritual practices, such as Indigenous Australians identifying with the 'mythical ancestors of the *alcheringa* period' and the rites of ancient Greece, Jung writes:

> This atavistic identification with human and animal ancestors can be interpreted psychologically as an integration of the unconscious, a veritable bath of renewal in the life-source where one is once again a fish, unconscious as in sleep, intoxication, and death. Hence the sleep of incubation, the Dionysian orgy, and the ritual death in initiation.
>
> (Jung 1980: 131)

In Jung's view, such opposition between consciousness and the unconscious is an inherent consequence of our species cognitive phylogeny, one that led to the development of very ancient forms of psychotherapy. For example, Jung calls the 'restitution ceremonies' of Indigenous Australians referred to in the above quote a form of psychotherapy that aims at individuation and integration of consciousness with the unconscious (Jung 2014a: 39–40). Elsewhere, he argues that psychology has yet to adequately understand 'the spiritual aspect of the psyche' which is known to us only in a very 'fragmentary way.' This unexplored and improperly understood aspect of human psychology is evident according to Jung in the 'spiritual processes of transformation in the psyche which underlie, for example, the well-known initiation rites of primitive peoples' (Jung 2014b: 462). Jung's approach helps us explain the neurophenomenology of altered states – that is both their experiential nature and their neurobiological substrates (Clark 2022). However, it is unlikely that an adaptationist account can explain the more nuanced subjective transformations involved in such states.

Robin Dunbar has explored these issues and postulated possible evolutionary explanations for trance or altered states. For example, commenting on Lewis Williams' research, he writes:

> Shamanic religions all over the world share a common set of motifs. These include entering the spirit world through a hole or tunnel beyond which there is an explosion of light and a bright world; all agree that travels in the spirit world are fraught with dangers that require a benign guide (either a well disposed ancestor or a totemic animal).
>
> (Dunbar 2014: 279)

In his commentary on this passage, Dunbar writes that religions 'seem to have evolved as a way of enhancing social cohesion and commitment within very small communities' in a manner that increases a sense of belonging to a community and typically makes people more generous towards each other' (Dunbar 2014: 280 and 82). While this is no doubt a valid assertion if we are thinking of religion as a form of sociality, it fails to account for the psychological nature of altered states of consciousness.

Tellingly, Dunbar acknowledges that trance dancers often collapse from exhaustion (Dunbar 2014: 279). It is hard to imagine why evolutionary processes selected for 'collapsing of exhaustion' as an adaptation. Collapsing during a state of trance suggests impaired functionality in some domains while others are enhanced.

The point is that there is something going on here that is psychological and not necessarily an evolved behaviour the genes for which have been selected over hundreds of thousands if not millions of years. Dunbar seems to get close to the nature of the problem in the following quote – but he fails to follow up the logic or implications of his own analysis:

> Among the San Bushmen of southern Africa, trance dances are particularly likely to take place when relationships within the extended community have started to unravel as people bicker among themselves. A trance dance restores the equilibrium, almost as though it wipes the slate clean of the toxic memories of the injustices and slights that poisoned relationships. Trance seems to reset relationships back to their default position, allowing the community to function once more as a mutually supportive network of relationships – until the petty slights and injustices build up again over the ensuing weeks and months, and a new trance dance is called for. This probably reflects the fact that trance dancing – if not the trance state itself – is associated with a massive release of endorphins, and it is these, acting in their time-honoured fashion to bond individuals, that make for restored relationships. In addition, endorphins have a widely beneficial effect on our physical and psychological health, and so trance dances likely benefit the health of the community as a whole, as well as its social cohesion.
>
> (Dunbar 2014: 279–80)

Dunbar hints at what a more nuanced psychological analysis might entail in his comments on wiping 'the slate clean of toxic memories.' The question is what exactly is being wiped clean? What are the associated changes in neural architecture? And how do these changes relate to uniquely human cognitive systems? As noted above, altered states of consciousness are associated with reduced activity in recently evolved neural hubs, desegregation of brain regions, ego dissolution and a shift to phylogenetically older core processes in the brain. Jung's conception of ritual as a process that seeks to integrate consciousness with more ancient brain systems not only explains the ritual Dunbar describes more effectively than Dunbar's own explanation; it is also supported by neuroscientific data.

The notion of wiping the 'slate clean' of 'toxic memories' suggests that the purpose of ritualised dance is to reconfigure the brain or to reboot it – which is what acute forms of altered consciousness often achieve (Carhart-Harris and Friston 2019). Because of his adaptationist orientation, Dunbar fails to see the problem in his analysis. If he did, I suspect he would appreciate that such behaviours are not so much adaptations but attempts to abrogate higher cognitive brain systems– which is what the concept of 'wiping the slate clean' implies. There is a paradox here: the more recently evolved cognitive adaptations that seemed to have led to our evolutionary success as a species may also be the cause of our psychological suffering – as was highlighted in the previous chapter in the discussion of Burns's book *The Descent of Madness* (Burns 2007*)*. Ritual and religion seem to have developed as technologies to address this evolutionary curse. Jung seems to have recognised this in his assertion that ritual life represents an ancient form of psychotherapy designed to integrate consciousness with the unconscious – that is the phylogenetically ancient socio-affective foundations of consciousness.

This evolutionary approach to the ethnographic record has more explanatory power than ones that explain ritual solely as an adaptation. There is a significant body of evidence in the anthropological literature that rituals – and particularly initiation rituals – are means by which humans seek to integrate more ancient brain systems with the more recently evolved forms of secondary consciousness associated with the ego complex. Moreover, such rituals often seek to obviate those more recently evolved brain systems, while activating evolutionarily older aspects of the brain. In this sense, Jung's approach seems to account for the ethnographic data, whereas adaptationist models fall short.

Initiation Rites and Adolescent Cognitive Development

In Chapter 4, I explored the evolution of an adolescent period of brain maturation as one of the distinguishing characteristics of our species. I highlighted how an extension of ontogeny over evolutionary time most likely underpinned the emergence of the default mode network and the uniquely human sense of self or ego. One crucial feature of this process, in both ontogeny and phylogeny, is that it seems to involve transition from subcortical primary process to secondary process modes of cognition. Crucially, during individual development or ontogeny, this transition takes place during adolescence – which is a uniquely human period of maturation.

Adolescent initiation rituals seem to be specifically designed to facilitate this transition. Initiation rites are common throughout the world, particularly in hunter-gatherer societies, where they mark the transition from childhood, through adolescence and into adulthood (van Gennep 1960; Stanner, Hogbin, and Beckett 1989; Cohen 2010). Among Australian hunter-gatherers, according to Stanner, such rites involve the subduing of 'youthful egotism so as to accord with the modes approved for men, and to bring some understanding to traditional mysteries.' Such a process is deployed in the ethical development of character, giving the initiates a sense of purpose 'beyond themselves, beyond egotism, and beyond social gain' bringing about a sense of 'unity that, however transient, was higher than any other occasions of social life made possible' (Stanner, Hogbin, and Beckett 1989: 299, 301 and 19).

Psychoactive compounds are a common feature of ritual life cross-culturally. Crucially, they also play an important role in adolescent initiation rites. There is evidence that Indigenous Australians use psychoactive plants for ritual purposes and the cultivation of altered states of consciousness, particularly in initiation rites where they help neophytes endure the austerities required for the attainment of manhood (de Rios and Stachalek 1999; Ratsch, Steadman, and Bogossian 2010). In Africa among the peoples of Gabon, the psychedelic plant Iboga is the central focus of sacramental Bwiti rituals. Significantly, one of the most important rites of passage facilitated by the Bwiti ceremonies is the transition through adolescence into adulthood (Goutarel 1993). Such use of psychedelics in initiation ceremonies is, according to Charles Grob and Marlene Dobkin de Rios, central to the promotion of prosocial behaviour as individuals transition from childhood to become members of the social group. As they write:

> In contrast to dangerous and irreverent use in contemporary society plant halluci-nogens were generally utilised by *Homo sapiens* within a ritualised, sacrosanct, socially sanctioned context with the intent to contribute to group cohesiveness and survival, particularly in pubertal initiatory rituals of identity. The unique suggestibility properties of the plants made them ideal catalysts of this process.
>
> (de Rios and Grob 1995: 115)

During the altered states induced by Iboga, participants experience a 'return to infancy and to birth – to the life in the womb.' Such a return to the 'uterine condi-tion' is believed to bring the individual 'very close to life in the land of the dead,' a sense of closeness which restores 'their own integrity – their pristine condition' (Fernandez 1982: 491). Significantly, the phenomenology of such experiences, like those of shamans mentioned by Dunbar, involve light, brightness or numinosity; as one of the chants used in the ceremonies indicates: 'Everything clean, clean. All is new, new. All is bright, bright. I have seen the dead and I do not fear' (Fernandez 1982: 488–9). Such rituals seem to produce an ontogenetic regression, in which the default mode network and neural hierarchies associated with ego consciousness collapse (Clark 2021: 16–8). Interestingly, the quality of consciousness resulting from the collapse of neural hierarchies under psychedelics has been likened to infancy and other spiritual states, such as those Wordsworth gave expression to in his poem on childhood, *Ode: Intimations of Immortality form Recollection of Early Childhood* (Brouwer and Carhart-Harris 2021: 337).

Benny Shanon has analysed the phenomenology of the psychedelic experience in his pioneering study *The Antipodes of the Mind: Charting the Phenomenology of the Ayahuasca Experience*. While its pharmacological profile is different, Aya-huasca is similar to LSD and psilocybin mushrooms in its effects. Shanon argues that the Ayahuasca experience is an example of an 'uncharted cognitive domain' yet to be fully investigated by cognitive science:

> The visions and other non-ordinary experiential phenomena that Ayahuasca in-duces present a new, uncharted natural cognitive domain. Since the number of natural domains is very small, this makes the Ayahuasca experience of para-mount interest for the student of mind … I am inclined to say that in various respects Ayahuasca brings us to the boundaries not only of science but also of the entire Western world view and its philosophies.
>
> (Shanon 2002: 34–35 and 39)

Jung was a pioneer explorer of this uncharted cognitive domain, decades ahead of his own times (Clark 2020, 2021). Since his passing, developments in the neuroscience of altered states of consciousness and the phenomenology of the psychedelic state, as well as an increasingly rich ethnographic record, have lent more and more credence to his ideas. The intellectual insularity of twentieth-century science, with its ethnocentric and monophasic assumptions about the human mind, has begun to ebb away in recent decades. The full significance of Jung's ideas is consequently becoming more apparent as the Enlightenment project of empirically based science begins exploring previously 'uncharted natural cognitive domains.' Such exploration represents individuation at the cultural and historical levels as human consciousness seeks to understand and integrate the deeper subcortical, unconscious layers of the mind into our scientific models of consciousness. As I have argued elsewhere, such a task, in terms of scientific investigation and the broader transformation of human culture and consciousness, is likely to become 'central to the future civilisational development of our species' (Clark 2022: 318–9 and 24–5).

Jung and Psychedelic Neuroscience

Psychedelic neuroscience has revolutionised our understanding of psychology and enabled researchers to study the deeper layers of the unconscious in laboratory settings – something that was particularly difficult in the past (Carhart-Harris et al. 2014). Psychedelics have the virtue of inducing 'ego dissolving' mystical experiences and profound forms of emotional catharsis reliably and predictably – consequently, such states can now be studied in an empirically rigorous manner (Carhart-Harris and Friston 2010; Nour et al. 2016). It is important when considering clinical applications that such experiences, in conjunction with supportive psychotherapy, have been shown to alleviate mental illness in ways previously not possible using more orthodox methods (Griffiths et al. 2006; MacLean, Johnson, and Griffiths 2011). This research paradigm also has significant implications for our understanding of brain evolution as well as developing new methods grounded in evolutionary neuroscience for the ethnographic analysis of psychedelic use in Indigenous cultures (Clark 2021, 2022).

Ethnographic data indicates the widespread cross-cultural use of psychedelics in sacred ritual contexts, with the archaeological record suggesting that they may have been part of human culture for centuries if not millennia (Adovasio and Fry 1976; Wasson 1980; Fernandez 1982; Terry et al. 2006; Ogalde, Arriaza, and Soto 2009; Beyer 2010). For example, there is evidence suggestive of psilocybin mushroom use going back some 7,000 years in Africa (Lajoux 1963; Samorini 2012; Clark 2021: 11–14). In Guatemala, mushroom stones, which are believed to have been associated with a hallucinogenic fertility cult, have been dated to between 6,000 and 2,000 years old (de Borhegyi 1961; Lowy 1971). An example of these stones is depicted in Figure 5.1.

It will be remembered from the above discussion that Jung saw ritual transformations of consciousness as a form of psychotherapy that aims at individuation and

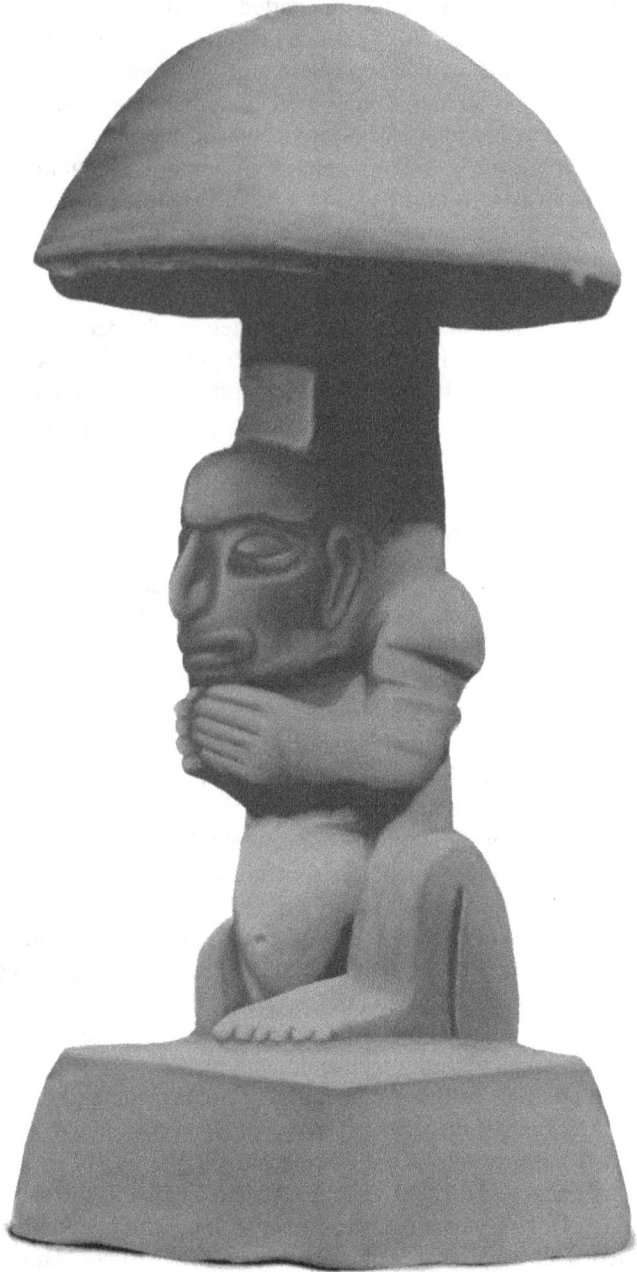

Figure 5.1 Guatemalan mushroom stone believed to be part of an ancient hallucinogenic fertility cult. Dated at approximately 1000 BC. Drawing adapted from Wasson (1980) by Matt Smale.

integration of consciousness with the unconscious (Jung 2014a: 39–40). It seems that the ritualised use of psychedelics in Indigenous cultures is similarly a very ancient form of therapy that produces quite profound psychological and somatic healing. For example, in her *Visionary Vine: Hallucinogenic Healing in the Peruvian Amazon*, Marlene Dobkin de Rois argues that traditional psychedelic-assisted healing 'represents a very old and honoured tradition of dealing with psychological problems that predates Freudian analysis by centuries' (de Rios 1984: 30).

Modern interest in the research and therapeutic potential of psychedelics was sparked by the synthesis of Lysergic acid diethylamide, commonly known as LSD, by the Swiss chemist Albert Hoffman in 1938 (Hofmann 2005). Consequent analysis by Hoffman confirmed the potential of LSD to alter the mind and body in ways previously unimagined (Hofmann 2005). Importantly, Hoffman analysed the LSD experience from the perspective of Freudian and Jungian psychology (Hofmann 2005: 53; Clark 2021: 3–4). During the 1950s and 1960s, consequent to Hofmann's discovery, more than a thousand scientific papers were published on psychedelic therapy, involving more than 40,000 research subjects, with many in the psychiatric establishment regarding the compounds as 'miracle drugs' (Pollan 2018: 3 and 44). During the 1960s and 1970s, this research programme came to an end, mostly due to political and cultural factors. They consequently became prohibited substances (Stevens 1987: 272–88).

Numerous writers during this early fertile period of research adopted Jungian perspectives in their approach to psychedelic-assisted therapy (Sandison 1954, 1959; Grof 1975). While Jung did not comment on psychedelic use in his writings, he did in a number of letters he wrote in the 1950s to the Dominican priest Victor White and to Betty Eisner, a psychologist who practised psychedelic-assisted psychotherapy in the 1950s and 1960s (Clark 2021: 4–7). In her letter to Jung, Eisner states that LSD is 'almost a religious drug' (Jung 1976: 382). In Jung's reply, he wrote:

> Experiments along the line of mescaline and related drugs are certainly most interesting, since such drugs lay bare a level of the unconscious that is otherwise accessible only under peculiar psychic conditions. It is a fact that you get certain perceptions and experiences of things appearing either in mystical states or in the analysis of unconscious phenomena, just like the primitives in their orgiastic or intoxicated conditions. I don't feel happy about these things, since you merely fall into such experiences without being able to integrate them.
>
> (Jung, Adler and Jaffé 1976: 382)

As the above comment illustrates, Jung's views on traditional psychedelic use seem to be expressive of his underlying ethnocentrism. Contemporary Jungian approaches to Indigenous use of psychedelics highlight the shortcomings of this aspect of Jung's thought while also emphasising the importance of his insights about psychedelics, the unconscious and individuation (Clark 2021: 5–7). Further, while Jung was sceptical of the irresponsible use of such compounds, contemporary researchers have refined Jung's approach and suggested that it is one that can be fruitfully employed in psychedelic-assisted therapies (Hill 2013; Carhart-Harris et al. 2014; Clark 2021).

In recent years, after decades of prohibition against psychedelic use in research and therapy, we have seen the emergence of a psychedelic renaissance (Sessa 2012; Pollan 2018). One of the pioneers in this field is Professor Robin Carhart-Harris who is currently the Director of the Neuroscape Psychedelics Division at the University of California. Carhart-Harris undertook some of the first neuroimaging studies of subjects who had been administered psychedelic compounds. Carhart Harris had a dual purpose in mind – to not only use psychedelics therapeutically to alleviate severe psychological suffering, but to also try and understand the neurobiology involved in such suffering. This research project also involved understanding how neural architecture is altered when such suffering is alleviated, and the mind begins to heal itself.

What is significant for analytical psychology is Carhart-Harris's belief that the phenomena manifested in the acute psychedelic state can be fruitfully explicated using Jung's theories. Carhart-Harris discusses the usefulness of William James' *The Varieties of Religious Experience* as a framework for explicating the psychedelic state – for example, James' notion that the unconscious is the source of mystical experience. For James, such states normally remain latent within the mind, yet may often become manifest in certain people; as he writes for '... persons deep in the religious life ... the door into this region seems unusually wide open.' Carhart-Harris quotes this passage approvingly, and the insights offered by James. He also discusses the relevance of Jung's evolutionary conception of the psyche to modern psychedelic research:

> Jung extended [James' ideas], arguing that the unconscious hosts the psychological remnants of our phylogenetic ancestry. In dreams, psychosis and other altered states, archetypal themes shaped by human history emerge into consciousness ... Jung's account of the "collective" unconscious fits comfortably with the phenomenology of the psychedelic experience. Archetypal themes feature heavily in user "trip reports" ... as they do in religious iconography.
>
> (Carhart-Harris et al. 2014: 14)

Carhart-Harris is of the opinion that psychedelics may help overcome the reticence among the scientific community in accepting the concept of the unconscious put forward by psychoanalysis. As he writes, reflecting on the inability to empirically demonstrate the existence of the unconscious, it is not 'surprising that with only dreaming and psychosis at its disposal, psychoanalysis has failed to convince the scientific community that the psychoanalytic unconscious exists.' As he elaborates:

> The unique scientific value of psychedelics rests in their capacity to make consciously accessible that which is latent in the mind ... mainstream psychology

and psychiatry have underappreciated the depth of the human mind by neglecting schools of thought that posit the existence of an unconscious mind. Indeed, psychedelics' greatest value may be as a remedy for ignorance of the unconscious mind.

(Carhart-Harris et al. 2014: 18)

Carhart-Harris is of the opinion that psychedelic research holds the potential for a revolutionary paradigm shift in our understanding of the mind and the therapeutic treatment of mental illness; as he writes 'for those brave enough to embrace it, research with psychedelics could herald the beginning of a new scientifically informed psychoanalysis that has the potential to influence modern psychology and psychiatry' (Carhart-Harris et al. 2014: 18). Carhart-Harris concludes his paper with two quotes from Jung to illustrate his point. The first is: 'He who would fathom the psyche must not confuse it with consciousness, else he veils from his own sight the object he wishes to explore'; the second: 'Man's worst sin is unconsciousness' (Jung quoted in Carhart-Harris et al. 2014: 18).

Signs of a paradigm shift, with cross-pollination between analytical psychology and psychedelic therapies, are evident in a newly emerging body of Jungian scholarship (Hill 2013; Swank 2020; Clark 2020, 2021, 2022; Stein and Corbett 2023). While this work involves a paradigm shift in Jungian psychology inspired by psychedelic therapies and neuroscience, it is hoped that the evolutionary model outlined in this book may also contribute to a greater appreciation of Jung's idea among evolutionary theorists, experimental neuroscientists and the increasing number of scholars conducting empirically based psychedelic research.

One of the fruitful avenues pursued by neuroscience and experimental psychedelic research is the investigation of shared mechanisms underlying the psychedelic state, dream mentation and psychoses (Brouwer and Carhart-Harris 2021). Some of the proposed mechanisms shared by such states include a phase transition from secondary consciousness and ego functions, to a more primary process style of cognition with increased cross-modular talk and global communication between neural networks resulting in a less segregated brain (Gattuso et al. 2023). This provides the suggestion that all of these phenomena may be related to the evolved segregation of the human brain – segregation which is obviated in each instance.

Significantly, not only do psychedelics seem to desegregate the brain; they also increase communication between different brain areas and reduce rigid thinking in higher order cortical regions associated with ego consciousness (Carhart-Harris and Friston 2019; Luppi et al. 2021; Daws et al. 2022). Psychedelics also induce alteration to the phenomenal sense of self through disintegration of the default mode and salience networks – an experience in which the representational fictions of an enduring Cartesian self are unbound (Letheby and Gerrans 2017). This suggests that Enlightenment rationalism, and the notion of the Cartesian self, can quite easily dissolve, giving rise to modes of awareness subserved by more ancient brain systems that for the most part lie outside of the conscious mind's very limited and circumscribed range of experience.

One of the more interesting findings of this research is the ability of psychedelics to alter personality structure in profound ways. As noted above, mystical experiences and ego dissolution are common components of the acute psychedelic state (Carhart-Harris et al. 2014; Tagliazucchi et al. 2016). Significantly, psychedelics seem to increase long-term measures of openness (MacLean, Johnson and Griffiths 2011; Nour, Evans, and Carhart-Harris 2017) with such increases in openness being more pronounced in subjects who scored higher on measures of mystical experience during the psychedelic session (MacLean, Johnson, and Griffiths 2011). Significantly, evidence suggests that psychedelic-induced ego dissolution positively predicts liberal political views, openness and nature relatedness, and negatively predicts authoritarian political views (Nour, Evans, and Carhart-Harris 2017). Such dissolution of ego consciousness also seems to be associated with increased sympathy, emotional empathy and prosocial attitudes towards others, as well as a greater sense of connection with the environment, both of which are believed to be underpinned by an alteration in the processing of the relation between self and other resulting in reduced egocentric socio-cognitive bias (Preller et al. 2016; Pokorny et al. 2017).

In Chapter 4, I discussed the evolution of the default mode network and that it may be related to the extension of hominin life history, delayed sexual maturation and evolution of an adolescent period of socio-cognitive development. Additionally, the larger brain size associated with such delayed maturation may also have given rise to increased modularity and segregation between brain regions (Striedter 2004: 10–11). The above discussion suggests that psychedelics may in fact be reversing the trajectory of cognitive evolution – and not just any aspect of cognition, but the recently evolved and uniquely human aspects of our neural architecture. Importantly, during Ayahuasca sessions, information flows from more ancient subcortical and visual brain regions seem to increase, suggesting that as upper cortical regions loosen their control over the rest of the brain, content from lower more ancient regions is able to emerge into awareness (Alonso et al. 2015; Dominguez-Clave et al. 2016). Such perturbation of neural architecture may explain the emotionally rich and potent visual imagery evident in altered states of consciousness such as those experienced during Ayahuasca visions as well as those depicted by Jung in the *Red Book* (Clark 2020).

References

Adovasio, J.M., and G.F. Fry. 1976. 'Prehistoric Psychotropic Drug Use in Northeastern Mexico and Trans-Pecos Texas', *Economic Botany*, 30: 94–96.

Alonso, J.F., S. Romero, M.A. Mananas, and J. Riba. 2015. 'Serotonergic Psychedelics Temporarily Modify Information Transfer in Humans', *International Journal of Neuropsychopharmacology*, 18: 1–9.

Beyer, S. 2010. *Singing to the Plants: A Guide to Mestizo Shamanism in the Upper Amazon* (University of New Mexico Press).

Bourguignon, E. 1973. *Religion, Altered States of Consciousness and Social Change* (Ohio State University Press (T)).

Brouwer, A., and R.L. Carhart-Harris. 2021. 'Pivotal Mental States', *Journal of Psychopharmacology*, 35: 319–52.

Burns, J. 2007. *The Descent of Madness: Evolutionary Origins of Psychosis and the Social Brain* (Taylor & Francis).

Carhart-Harris, R.L., and K.J. Friston. 2010. 'The Default-Mode, Ego-Functions and Free-Energy: A Neurobiological Account of Freudian Ideas', *Brain*, 133: 1265–83.

Carhart-Harris, R.L., and K.J. Friston. 2019. 'REBUS and the Anarchic Brain: Toward a Unified Model of the Brain Action of Psychedelics', *Pharmacological Reviews*, 71: 316.

Carhart-Harris, R.L., R. Leech, P.J. Hellyer, M. Shanahan, A. Feilding, E. Tagliazucchi, et al. 2014. 'The Entropic Brain: A Theory of Conscious States Informed by Neuroimaging Research with Psychedelic Drugs', *Frontiers in Human Neuroscience*, 8: 149–64.

Clark, G. 2020. 'Integrating the Archaic and the Modern: The Red Book, Visual Cognitive Modalities and the Neuroscience of Altered States of Consciousness.' in Stein M., and T. Arzt (eds.), *Jung's Red Book for Our Time: Searching for Soul under Postmodern Conditions* (Chiron Publications).

Clark, G. 2021. 'Carl Jung and the Psychedelic Brain: An Evolutionary Model of Analytical Psychology Informed by Psychedelic Neuroscience', *International Journal of Jungian Studies*, 4(2): 1–30.

Clark, G. 2022. 'The Dionysian Primate: Goethe, Nietzsche, Jung and Psychedelic Neuroscience.' in Miils, J., and D. Burston (eds.), *Psychoanalysis and the Mind-Body Problem* (Routledge).

Clottes, J. 2009. 'Foreword.' in *Cave Paintings and the Human Spirit: The Origin of Creativity and Belief* (Prometheus Books).

Cohen, Y.A. 2010. *Legal Systems & Incest Taboos: The Transition from Childhood to Adolescence* (Aldine Transaction).

Daws, R.E., C. Timmermann, B. Giribaldi, J.D. Sexton, M.B. Wall, D. Erritzoe, et al. 2022. 'Increased Global Integration in the Brain after Psilocybin Therapy for Depression', *Nature Medicine*, 28: 844–51.

de Borhegyi, S. 1961. 'Miniature Mushroom Stones from Guatemala', *American Antiquity*, 26: 498–504.

de Rois, M.D., and C. Grob 1995. 'Hallucinogens, Suggestibility & Adolescence in Cross-Cultural Perspective', *Verlg Fur Wissenschaft und Bildung*, 22(1): 121–38.

de Rios, M.D., and R. Stachalek. 1999. 'The Duboisia Genus, Australian Aborigines and Suggestibility', *Journal of Psychoactive Drugs*, 31: 155–61.

de Rios, M.D. 1984. *Visionary Vine: Hallucinogenic Healing in the Peruvian Amazon* (Waveland Press).

Dominguez-Clave, E., J. Soler, M. Elices, J.C. Pascual, E. Alvarez, M. de la Fuente Revenga, et al. 2016. 'Ayahuasca: Pharmacology, Neuroscience and Therapeutic Potential', *Brain Research Bulletin*, 126: 89–101.

Dunbar, R. 2014. *Human Evolution: A Pelican Introduction* (Penguin Books Limited).

Fernandez, J.W. 1982. *Bwiti: An Ethnography of the Religious Imagination in Africa* (Princeton University Press).

Fink, B., B. Bläsing, A. Ravignani, and T. Shackelford. 2021. 'Evolution and Functions of Human Dance', *Evolution and Human Behavior*, 42: 351–60.

Flor-Henry, P., Y. Shapiro, C. Sombrun, and P. Walla. 2017. 'Brain Changes during a Shamanic Trance: Altered Modes of Consciousness, Hemispheric Laterality, and Systemic Psychobiology', *Cogent Psychology*, 4: 1313522.

Gattuso, J.J., D. Perkins, S. Ruffell, A.J. Lawrence, D. Hoyer, L.H. Jacobson, et al. 2023. 'Default Mode Network Modulation by Psychedelics: A Systematic Review', *International Journal of Neuropsychopharmacology*, 26: 155–88.

Goutarel, R. 1993. 'Pharmacodynamie et applications therapeutiques de l'iboga et de l'ibogaine', *Psychedelic Monographs and Essays*, 6: 70–111.

Griffiths, R.R., W.A. Richards, U. McCann, and R. Jesse. 2006. 'Psilocybin Can Occasion Mystical-Type Experiences Having Substantial and Sustained Personal Meaning and Spiritual Significance', *Psychopharmacology (Berl)*, 187: 268–83; discussion 84–92.

Grof, S. 1975. *Realms of the Human Unconscious: Observations from LSD Research* (Viking Press).

Hill, S.J. 2013. *Confrontation with the Unconscious: Jungian Depth Psychology and Psychedelic Experience* (Muswell Hill Press).

Hofmann, A. 2005. *LSD, My Problem Child: Reflections on Sacred Drugs, Mysticism, and Science* (Multidisciplinary Association for Psychedelic Studies).

Jung, C.G. 1953. *Collected Works of C. G. Jung, Volume 13: Alchemical Studies* (Princeton University Press).

Jung, C.G. 1976. *Letters* (Princeton University Press).

Jung, C.G. 1980. *Collected Works of C.G. Jung, Volume 12: Psychology and Alchemy* (Princeton University Press).

Jung, C.G. 2014a. *Collected Works of C.G. Jung, Volume 9 (Part 1): Archetypes and the Collective Unconscious* (Princeton University Press).

Jung, C.G. 2014b. *The Structure and Dynamics of the Psyche* (Taylor & Francis).

Jung, C.G., G. Adler, and A. Jaffé. 1976. *Letters* (Routledge).

Lajoux, J.D. 1963. *The Rock Paintings of Tassili* (World Publishing Company).

Laughlin, C.D. 2011. *Communing with the Gods: Consciousness, Culture and the Dreaming Brain* (Daily Grail Publishing).

Laughlin, C.D., J. McManus, and E.G. D'Aquili. 1990. *Brain, Symbol & Experience: Toward a Neurophenomenology of Human Consciousness* (New Science Library).

Letheby, C., and P. Gerrans. 2017. 'Self Unbound: Ego Dissolution in Psychedelic Experience', *Neuroscience of Consciousness*, 2017: nix016.

Lewis-Williams, D. 2004. *The Mind in the Cave: Consciousness and the Origins of Art* (Thames & Hudson).

Lewis-Williams, D., and S. Challis. 2011. *Deciphering Ancient Minds: The Mystery of San Bushman Rock Art* (Thames & Hudson).

Lowy, B. 1971. 'New Records of Mushroom Stones from Guatemala, *Mycologia*, 63(5): 983–93.

Luppi, A.I., R.L. Carhart-Harris, L. Roseman, I. Pappas, D.K. Menon, and E.A. Stamatakis. 2021. 'LSD Alters Dynamic Integration and Segregation in the Human Brain', *NeuroImage*, 227: 117653.

MacLean, K.A., M.W. Johnson, and R.R. Griffiths. 2011. 'Mystical Experiences Occasioned by the Hallucinogen Psilocybin Lead to Increases in the Personality Domain of Openness', *Journal of Psychopharmacology*, 25: 1453–61.

Nietzsche, F. 1994. *Human, All Too Human* (Penguin Books Limited).

Nour, M.M., L. Evans, and R.L. Carhart-Harris. 2017. 'Psychedelics, Personality and Political Perspectives', *Journal of Psychoactive Drugs*, 49: 182–91.

Nour, M.M., L. Evans, D. Nutt, and R.L. Carhart-Harris. 2016. 'Ego-Dissolution and Psychedelics: Validation of the Ego-Dissolution Inventory (EDI)', *Frontiers in Human Neuroscience*, 10: 467–72.

Ogalde, J.P., B.T. Arriaza, and E.C. Soto. 2009. 'Identification of Psychoactive Alkaloids in Ancient Andean Human Hair by Gas Chromatography/Mass Spectrometry', *Journal of Archaeological Science*, 36: 467–72.

Pokorny, T., K.H. Preller, M. Kometer, I. Dziobek, and F.X. Vollenweider. 2017. 'Effect of Psilocybin on Empathy and Moral Decision-Making', *International Journal of Neuropsychopharmacology*, 20: 747–57.

Pollan, M. 2018. *How to Change Your Mind: What the New Science of Psychedelics Teaches Us about Consciousness, Dying, Addiction, Depression, and Transcendence* (Penguin Publishing Group).

Preller, K.H., T. Pokorny, A. Hock, R. Kraehenmann, P. Stämpfli, E. Seifritz, et al. 2016. 'Effects of Serotonin 2A/1A Receptor Stimulation on Social Exclusion Processing', *Proceedings of the National Academy of Sciences*, 113: 5119–24.

Ratsch, A., K.J. Steadman, and F. Bogossian. 2010. 'The Pituri Story: A Review of the Historical Literature Surrounding Traditional Australian Aboriginal Use of Nicotine in Central Australia', *Journal of Ethnobiology and Ethnomedicine*, 6: 26.

Samorini. 2012. 'Mushroom Effigies in World Archaeology: From Rock Art to Mushroom-Stones', *Proceedings of the Conference "The stone mushrooms of Thrace", Greek Open University, Alexandroupolis*, 16–42.

Sandison, R.A. 1954. 'Psychological Aspects of the Lsd Treatment of the Neuroses', *Journal of Mental Science*, 100: 508–15.

Sandison, R.A. 1959. 'The Role of Psychotropic Drugs in Individual Therapy', *Bulletin of the World Health Organization*, 21: 495–503.

Sessa, B. 2012. *The Psychedelic Renaissance: Reassessing the Role of Psychedelic Drugs in 21st Century Psychiatry and Society* (Muswell Hill Press).

Shanon, B. 2002. *The Antipodes of the Mind: Charting the Phenomenology of the Ayahuasca Experience* (Oxford University Press).

Stanner, W.E.H., H.I. Hogbin, and J. Beckett. 1989. *On Aboriginal Religion* (University of Sydney).

Stein, L., and L. Corbett. 2023. *Psychedelics and Individuation: Essays by Jungian Analysts* (Chiron Publications).

Stevens, J. 1987. *Storming Heaven: LSD and the American Dream* (Grove Press).

Striedter, G.F. 2004. *Brain Evolution* (Sinauer).

Swank, M. 2020. 'Mercurius Ubiquitous: A Jungian Approach to Psychedelic Therapy', *International Journal of Jungian Studies*, 13: 13–40.

Tagliazucchi, E., L. Roseman, M. Kaelen, C. Orban, S.D. Muthukumaraswamy, K. Murphy, et al. 2016. 'Increased Global Functional Connectivity Correlates with LSD-Induced Ego Dissolution', *Current Biology*, 26: 1043–50.

Terry, M., K.L. Steelman, T. Guilderson, P. Dering, and M.W. Rowe. 2006. 'Lower Pecos and Coahuila Peyote: New Radiocarbon Dates', *Journal of Archaeological Science*, 33: 1017–21.

van Gennep, A. 1960. *The Rites of Passage* (Routledge).

Wasson, R.G. 1980. *The Wondrous Mushroom: Mycolatry in Mesoamerica* (McGraw-Hill).

Whitley, D.S. 2009. *Cave Paintings and the Human Spirit: The Origin of Creativity and Belief* (Prometheus Books).

Wilson, D. 2003. *Darwin's Cathedral: Evolution, Religion, and the Nature of Society* (University of Chicago Press).

Winkelman, M. 2010. *Shamanism: A Biopsychosocial Paradigm of Consciousness and Healing* (Praeger).

Winkelman, M. 2017. 'The Mechanisms of Psychedelic Visionary Experiences: Hypotheses from Evolutionary Psychology', *Frontiers in Neuroscience*, 11: 1–17.

Chapter 6

Anthropology and Analytical Psychology

Introduction

As discussed in Chapter 2, Jung was influenced by the concept of the Dreaming as it was articulated by Spencer and Gillen. In that chapter, I argued that the similarities between Jung's thought and French sociology, and particularly that of Durkheim, were due in large part to their reliance on the same ethnographic sources. In this chapter, I explore those issues in more detail, linking concepts of the sacred, blood symbolism, exogamy, sexual politics and the Dreaming. I will explore similar concepts in African and Australian hunter-gatherer societies, which, given their temporal and geographic separation, suggests that both cultures derive from a very ancient source culture with a shared underlying neurobiology and social structure. The differences between these cultures also highlight how societies may vary, while still giving expression to underlying archetypal motifs and ritual practices. In this chapter, the various threads of previous chapters are woven together providing a kind summation and demonstration of the explanatory utility of the model in regard to the ethnographic literature.

First Creation and Healing Sickness

Ritual among the San of Africa, also known as the !Kung, exhibits certain important features of neurobiology explored in this book. These include what appears to be deactivation of higher cortical brain centres as well as blood symbolism. During periodic gatherings for ritual events, extended dancing occurs with participants entering trance and young people often being initiated (Lee 1979: 366–7). Important occasions for such ritual activity are when 'male youths begin to hunt seriously and girls to menstruate' (Finnegan 2013: 705). Additionally, as Power notes when commenting on such ethnographic data, 'women use idioms of bleeding together to express connection and belonging' (Power 2022: 10).

As already noted in previous chapters, one of the important purposes of ritual is to alter consciousness, which is often achieved through all-night singing and dancing sessions. Modern ethnographies which describe such processes provide

DOI: 10.4324/9781032624549-7

support for Jung's notion that ritual is an ancient form of psychotherapy in which more recently evolved brain regions go into abeyance. For example, in their paper 'Reentry into First Creation,' Hillary and Bradford Keeney argue that the ritual gatherings of the !Kung involve the loss of conscious control:

> Their singing is inspired improvisation that triggers additional body automatisms, the effortless trembling that feels as if the mind has less conscious control over one's performance. Narrating and evaluating mind give way to improvised spontaneous movements, rhythm, and music. More aesthetic engagement with others is fostered, resulting in interactions that aim to inspire healing and transformation.
>
> (Keeney and Keeney 2013: 78)

The !Kung believe that existence is divided into two domains: First Creation, a time in the past when people could 'change into animals, communicate with all living forms, and have eternal life without sickness' and Second Creation, which represents the condition of current humans (Keeney and Keeney 2013: 65). Ritual is a means of transitioning from Second Creation back into First Creation – a transformation that may be effected by participants wearing ritual regalia in which they play the role of animals, or of actual transformations of consciousness. Significantly, Jung argued that such ritual transformation into animals represents an ancient form of psychotherapy; as he writes, 'atavistic identification with human and animal ancestors can be interpreted psychologically as an integration of the unconscious' (Jung 1980: 131).

Such ritual activates a form of energy in the lower abdominal regions the !Kung refer to as n/om. Activation of lower abdominal regions suggests that higher cortical regions associated with ego consciousness are deactivated. In his book *Boiling Energy: Community Healing Among the Kalahari Kung*, Richard Katz analyses the way in which n/om or 'boiling energy' is activated during ritual. One of the main functions of !Kung ritual is to heal physical and psychological sickness. As Katz writes: 'Sickness is more an existential condition or level of being than a particular illness or symptom. Everybody has some sickness, and so everybody who is at a dance is given healing' (Katz 1982: 102). Boiling energy or n/om enables participants to 'heal or pull out sickness.' When entering such states, participants transition beyond their 'ordinary level of experience' and report having 'nothing in [their] head' (Katz 1982: 42).

The climax of !Kung ritual involves the experience of an enhanced state of consciousness referred to as !*kia* which results from n/om rising up the central axis of the spine to the base of the skull. This movement of energy up the spinal cord during trance has been compared to *Kundalini* yoga which seeks to release energies in the base of the spine enabling them to travel up through the heart and crown of the head (Hume 2002: 58–9). As I discuss below, similar comparisons between yoga and Aboriginal Australian medicine men have also been suggested.

One informant described to Katz the nature of this emptying out or purifying of consciousness: 'I want to have a dance again so I can really become myself' (Katz 1982: 43). Such alterations of consciousness also have a positive impact in promoting prosocial emotions such as forgiveness and open heartedness. As one informant told Keeney: 'Everyone who goes to the ceremony gets an open heart and feels good about the community, even forgiving someone who stole his wife' (Keeney 2000: 63). Interestingly, particularly in the past, the attainment of such altered or enriched states of consciousness was facilitated by the use of psychedelic compounds (Winkelman and Dobkin de Rios 1989) which were thought to result in a much more intense and stronger alteration of consciousness during ritualised dancing and singing among the !Kung (Katz 1982: 284; Clark 2017). Such use seems to be less common among contemporary !Kung.

It is clear from the above discussion that the purpose of !Kung ritual is to deactivate higher cognitive centres associated with narration, evaluation and upper cortical thought processes. When such aspects of neural architecture go into abeyance, emotions such as forgiveness and openheartedness pervade social life. This field data provides a demonstration of the utility of the model outlined in this book. For example, cognitive centres associated with the default mode network and ego consciousness are known to be involved in the creation of autobiographical narratives, internal cognitive rumination and associated forms of psychopathology (Spreng, Mar, and Kim 2008; Carhart-Harris et al. 2014; Carhart-Harris and Friston 2019; Zhou et al. 2020). Curing 'sickness' by having 'nothing' in one's 'head,' having less 'conscious control' and reducing the activity of the 'narrating and evaluating mind' all seem to suggest deactivation of this network. This does suggest that such rituals, as has been noted in neuroimaging studies of shamanic trance and altered states of consciousness, effect desegregation of brain regions, ego dissolution, a shift to phylogenetically older core processes and an associated phase transition from recently evolved secondary process to primary process affective systems (Flor-Henry et al. 2017; Carhart-Harris and Friston 2019; Luppi et al. 2021; Daws et al. 2022: 20). Importantly, altered states of consciousness have also been shown to increase empathy and decrease egocentric socio-cognitive bias (Preller et al. 2016; Pokorny et al. 2017). These alterations of neural architecture most likely underpin the claims of the !Kung that ritual facilitates forgiveness and openheartedness.

As I noted in Chapter 5 in my discussion of Dunbar's thoughts on the evolution of religion (Dunbar 2014: 279–82), it is unlikely that the above behaviours are the result of cognitive adaptations that have been favoured over millennia by natural selection – i.e., it is doubtful that they are components of the species specific human genome. This is because such activities are explicitly about deactivating higher cognitive centres, reactivating visceral and affective responses and entering out of the everyday human world and back into the world of First Creation. Given these activities seem to involve deactivation of recently evolved brain areas, it is hard to see them as having evolved through natural selection. They are most likely cultural technologies that seek to integrate inadequately integrated brain systems – i.e., they are an ancient form of psychotherapy with the aim being individuation as Jung argued. As noted in Chapter 5, orthodox evolutionary accounts seem unable to account for the experiential nature of human ritual life and the phenomena of altered states of consciousness. The model of analytical psychology informed by evolutionary science and life history theory outlined in this book seems much more adequate to the task of explicating such cultural phenomena than orthodox adaptationist models of ritual and religion.

Dreams, Culture and the Unconscious

As noted in Chapter 5, dreams have been long proposed as the source of supernatural beliefs by theorists such as Edward Tylor (1832–1917), Frederick Netizsche (1844–1900) and Jung. This theory is supported by extensive cross-cultural data where dreams are believed to be the source of supernatural agent concepts (Lincoln 1970; McNamara and Bulkeley 2015; Bulkeley 2016). While Indigenous cultures distinguish between dreamlife and waking reality, it is not uncommon for them to consider 'dream experience' as having 'greater reality value than an actual experience' (Lincoln 1970: 28). This belief is very common in Indigenous Australian cultures and is inherent in the concept of the Dreaming (Hume 2002: 24–37). While there are differences between African and Australian cultures and ritual, there are also similarities. These mostly involve inducement of altered states and reversion to primary process modes of cognition.

In order to give some idea of what the term conveys to Indigenous people themselves, I quote the following from the Pitjantjatjara women Nganyinytja. Nganyinytja was born in Central Australia in 1928 and during her childhood, she had very little direct contact with white people. The following description is from the book that accompanied the 2014 Ngintaka exhibition at the South Australian Museum. The exhibition was an Indigenous-led project that sought to showcase to the wider Australian public Central Australian Dreaming stories and sacred sites about Ngintaka, the ancestral Perentie Lizard or Sand Goanna. This is how Nganyinytja describes her early education in the desert:

> We have no books, our history was not written by people with pen and paper. It is in the land, the footprints of our Creation Ancestors are on the rocks … We learned from our grandmothers and grandfathers as they showed us these sacred sites, told us the stories, sang and danced with us the Tjukurpa (the Law or Dreaming). We remember it all, in our minds, our bodies and feet as we dance the stories. We continually recreate the Tjukurpa … The land is our school. We learn to read where the Ancestors have moved through this country, where they have created the foods that we now gather, they are responsible for the animals that we now hunt. This has been our school and that's how I grew up, that's what I was learning to read, the Law, the creation stories of the land. This land is alive with the stories of the Rainbow Serpent and the Sand Goanna and all the Creation Beings who came through here. Our families have kept these alive.
>
> (Nganyinytja quoted in James et al. 2014: 15–6)

When we take the Indigenous perspective into account, Jung's notion of dream-life as the font of religion and spirituality seems to be in many essential senses correct. Anthropologist W.H. Stanner has expressed a view that is consilient with Jung's view; as he writes in his discussion of the concept of the Dreaming, there is

> ... an implicit theory of something very like the unconscious ... That is, a theory that elemental forces, antecedent to the formation of the mature human being in society, operate below the level of the waking or conscious mind by continuing perennially through sleep and dream, as major determinants of conscious human conduct.
>
> (Stanner 1998: 7)

Nancy Munn's 1973 *Walbiri Iconography: Graphic Representation and Cultural Symbolism in a Central Australian Society* provides ethnographic insights that are germane to the evolutionary model of analytical psychology outlined in this book. Munn is an American anthropologist who carried out field work in the 1950s among the Walbiri people of Yuendumu, a Western Desert community about 200 kilometres west of Alice Springs. Munn's field work highlights the important role of sex-based categories in Walbiri social and religious life, with strict demarcation between men's and women's 'business.' The rituals of men and women have distinct functions; women focus more on 'growing up' or nurturing the immediate family, while men's rituals are designed to ensure the fertility of the ecosystems and the continuation of the cosmos as a whole. However, these domains intersect as the performance of male fertility rites also ensure the land is able to sustain their community and hence ensure women are able to successfully perform their social roles.

Munn explains this distinction as between 'masculine symbolic or social creativity, and feminine, biological creativity' (Munn 1973: 209). This binary system is evident in the designs used in ritual which distinguish between icons of camp (circles denoting female) and hunting paths or tracks (lines denoting male). Such 'binary oppositions,' writes Munn, constitute 'the dominant symbolism' of ritual life. However, this opposition is part of a dualistic system of 'complementarity and polarization' that on another level constitutes wholeness or social unity (Munn 1973: 220).

This sense of symbolic complementarity is evident in the manner in which male and female symbolism inform one another in the ritual domain. For example, *churingas* such as boards or stones are coated in ochre (Munn 1973: 50–1) which establishes associations with blood, the sacred and the female domain of existence. Male dancers may also have designs painted on their body representing both male and female iconographies; as Munn writes, the dancer may be 'decked out in forms representing both female and male elements, the camp and the path expressed in the combination of circular headdress and linear body designs' (Munn 1973: 50–1).

Central to both sexes however is the dynamic between two different levels of reality that become manifest in dreamlife and ritual. For example, for the Warlpiri, existence is divided into two realms, that of *djugurba* and *yidjaru*. *Djugurba* refers to the abstract creative period that Nganyinytja was referring to above in her description of the Dreaming (spelt *tjukurpa* in the Pitjantjatjara language). *Djugurba* is also linked with sleep and dreamlife. *Yidjaru* however refers to actual individual people living in the here and now, that is the realm of waking individualised consciousness, a realm which is distinct from dreamlife and sleep and their association with the ancestral creative period. These terms correspond to Jung's ego consciousness and the collective unconscious – in fact, they could be used instead of *djugurba* and *yidjaru* without any real loss of meaning. Additionally, Jung's concept of a 'split psyche' consisting of antagonism between consciousness and the collective unconscious – an antagonism that humans seek to heal through ritual – provides a robust evolutionary explanation of the phenomenology of ritual experience (Jung 2014b: 253–64).

For the Walpiri, the membrane separating *djugurba* and *yidjaru* is permeable. Further, it is through dreamlife and ritual that the realm of *djugurba* emerges into the realm of *yidjaru*. In a sense, ritual becomes an inversion of reality, where the hidden dimension of dreamlife becomes manifest in concrete form in the field of waking sensory perception. In normal waking consciousness dreamlife, and its association with the creative period or Dreaming, is hidden. However, when the dancer dresses in the ceremonial regalia of his or her ancestor, that hidden dimension is now manifest in the realm of waking reality. That is, the everyday waking self is now itself hidden underneath the ceremonial representation of the performer's totemic ancestor. As Munn writes:

Through the designs and songs the sense of values and tradition bound up with the notion of *djgurba* 'surfaces' or becomes publicly visible, and so is integrated into the perceptual field and sense experience of the social world of waking reality ... Dreams and rite constitute complementary poles of a single process. The dream works in a private consciousness of sleep, while the ceremonial works in the waking rational order of the social world; both structure the relation between actor and event in a different way from that of ordinary experience, for in the latter the subjective integration of the individual with the 'cut-off' *djugurba* range of experience is not central, while in dreams and ceremony this is the key feature.

(Munn 1973: 103)

Walpiri thought, and particularly as outlined by Munn, is strikingly similar to Jung's conception of a deep layer in the psyche that lay hidden from consciousness – or in Jung's terminology split off or dissociated. Further, Jung's theory that ritual involves the integration of the collective unconscious with consciousness seems to be exactly what we see occurring in Walpiri ritual. Of course, the terminology is different – but the underlying process being described is the same. For example, in

Jung's theory, we could quite easily replace collective unconscious and consciousness with *djugurba* and *yidjaru* and his meaning would be retained.

It is important to note that while the phrase the Dreaming is derived from English, Aboriginal people themselves use it to describe stories of the land's creation and aspects of totemic geography and associated kinship rules and forms of land tenure. Again, this concept has strong affinities with Jung's theory of the collective unconscious; to quote anthropologist W.E.H. Stanner:

> Evidently the use of the English word (which is in universal currency from Central Australia to North Australia, and doubtless has passed from tribe to tribe) is an attempt, by metaphor based on analogy, to convey the mystical quality of the relations as being like the relation of dream-life to waking-life. At the same time one must note that, to the Aborigines, an actual dream-experience is agentive and prophetic. Their choice of the English word seems to me a brilliant economy of phrase, covering both the denotations and connotations of the mystical conception of totemism within the ontology.
>
> (Stanner 2014: 26)

I have only touched on what is a rich and fertile area for Jungians to explore, bringing together sensitive cultural analysis with models of analytical psychology informed by evolutionary neuroscience.

Archetypal Variations: Blood Symbolism and Sexual Politics

Some of the most important components of human culture are blood symbolism and serpent imagery. Blood symbolism was discussed in Chapter 2 and links with female reproduction and lunar cycles were highlighted. In that chapter, I discussed how this was an important concern for Jungian scholars going back to Esther Harding's writing in the 1930s, to the more recent work of Erich Neuman and Sylvia Perera (Harding 1936; Perera 1981; Neumann 1994). I also noted the association between female reproductive cycles, lunar cycles and menstruation in Indigenous cultures.

Blood symbolism exists in both African and Australian foraging societies, whose cultures evolved vast distances from one another and which have been separated for tens of thousands of years. This suggests that such symbolism, and the associated mythological systems, may represent a source cosmology for our species (Power 2017). Commenting on similar symbolism in Africa and Australia, archaeologist Ian Watts writes that 'something like a Rainbow Serpent-type creature' may have been 'part of the symbolic template of early *Homo sapiens*, an elaboration of the logic informing the world's first metaphor—equating women's blood with the blood of game animals' (Watts 2017: 263).

Chris Knight argues that the Australian Rainbow Serpent is a variation on a global theme, an image that encapsulates metamorphosis, change and cyclical time: in the Australian context the time of the wet and dry seasons, the 'wet' period of menstruation and the endogamous tendency of close familial bonds which is the antithesis and opposite of exogamous marriage outside the group (Knight 1988). He quotes Marshack to illustrate his point: 'the serpent of time, of process and continuity, the serpent of self-birth and origins, the serpent of death, birth, and rebirth, the cosmic serpent, the serpent of such processes as water, rain, and lightning, the ouroboros that bites its own tail in perpetuity, the guilloche serpent of endless continuity and turns' (Marshack 1985: 142). Commenting on this passage, Knight observes that 'Snake symbolism in Australia, as elsewhere, is associated with the innermost mysteries of secret rites and cults' (Knight 1988: 243).

In analytical psychology, the association between serpent imagery and the feminine is frequently commented upon. For example, Jung associated serpent imagery with the anima archetype also noting that the yogic Kundalini serpent, which is believed to reside in the abdominal cavity at the base of spine, also resides in caves or the womb of the earth (Jung 2014a: 200, 2014d: 436). Neumann also commented on snakes as the consort of The Great Mother (Neumann 1954: 48–9). The prevalence of serpent imagery in psychedelic visions, their possible neurobiological substrates and their centrality to Jungian psychology has been explored in detail by Hereward Tilton in his excellent *The Path of the Serpent: Psychedelics and the Neuropsychology of Gnosis* (Tilton 2020; Clark 2022).

In his discussion of these issues, Knight recounts the myth of the Wawilak Sisters, a Dreaming story from Arnhem Land in Northern Australia. This story highlights how menstrual blood and initiation rituals are interconnected. It recounts the association between two sisters, the Rainbow Snake who resides in a waterhole and how the two sisters taught men how to perform sacred rituals. For example, the blood that is used in ritual is believed to be derived from the women. Importantly, women's menstrual cycles seem to be associated with incestuous relationships among the mythical sisters – which evokes the endogamous coalitions of women mentioned by Finnegan in her description of female dance and ritual in Chapter 3. As Knight writes, when commenting on the mythological theme of being swallowed and regurgitated by the Rainbow Snake, and how this relates to menstrual taboos and seclusion:

> Assuming that menstrual blood is thought of as "wet" rather than "dry," menstrual seclusion should be depictable as a snake's drawing of women into a watery world. In terms of detailed mythological imagery, the "swallowing" episodes would be associated with pools, streams, marshes, rains, storms, wet season, and so on, while the "regurgitations" would be linked with dryness (fire, dry earth, sun, dry season, etc.) ... Menstrual seclusion in the real world is a withdrawal from exogamous sex into "one's own blood," so no union with a snake should have the characteristics of legitimate exogamous marriage. Snake marriage should be a union of blood with blood—that is, an intimacy comparable with the incestuous relationships of the Wawilak Sisters.
>
> (Knight 1988: 247)

We can see here an example in mythic form of the female coalitionary dances and rituals performed by African women mentioned in Chapter 3 – what Finnegan called 'ritual celebrations of reproductive sex, birth, blood, and the female genitals' (Finnegan 2013: 707). In numerous Australian Indigenous cultures, this archetypal material seems to have been appropriated from the female domain and used in the male domain. This represents an example of variation on an archetypal motif that associates blood with sacredness, the feminine and rebirth. But in this instance, it is transformation of male psychology utilising imagery derived from female reproductive biology. Knight quotes from the anthropologist Warner who highlights this process. Warner was told by an Indigenous informant how the Wawilak Sisters myth relates to male ritual:

> That blood we put all over those men is all the same as the blood that came from that old woman's vagina. It isn't the blood of those men any more because it has been sung over and made strong. The hole in the man's arm isn't that hole any more. It is all the same as the vagina of that old woman that had blood coming out of it.
>
> (Warner 1969: 268)

Knight highlights the frequently reported opinion of Aboriginal men that the use of blood in male sacred rituals originally came from women – in fact that men stole the ritual practice from women. Knight cites such an account by an Aboriginal man quoted from the Berndt's study of sexual behaviour in Western Arnhem Land:

> But really we have been stealing what belongs to them (the women), for it is mostly all women's business; and since it concerns them it belongs to them. Men have nothing to do really, except copulate, it belongs to the women. All that belonging to those Wuwalak, the baby, the blood, the yelling, their dancing, all that concerns the women; but every time we have to trick them. Women can't see what men are doing, although it really is their own business, but we can see their side. This is because all the Dreaming business came out of women— everything; only men take "picture" for that Julunggul [i.e., men make an artificial reproduction of the Snake]. In the beginning we had nothing, because men had been doing nothing; we took these things from women.
>
> (Berndt and Berndt 1951: 55)

These observations have implications for cross-cultural sexual politics and symbolism of blood and birth derived from female reproductive capacity. Among small-scale, immediate return hunter-gatherers, numerous Indigenous Australian societies are distinguished by a relative absence of egalitarian relations between the sexes. It is true that women in these societies possess important roles in terms or ritual and cultural life and wield significant power especially as they age (Dussart 2000; Bell 2002: 240). However, the sexual politics of such societies are very different from those of more sex-egalitarian African foragers (Shostak 2009: 220–1;

Konner 2015: 141). For example, numerous Indigenous Australian societies have a significant bias towards patriarchal social structures and culturally sanctioned subordination and control of women's sexuality and reproductive capacity (Meggitt 1962: 90 and 91; Bell and Nelson 1989; Kimm 2004; Sutton 2005; Clark 2014).

Commenting on this aspect of Australian Indigenous culture, Knight argues, in agreement with the Aboriginal men quoted above, that the ritual use of blood or its symbolic equivalent such as ochre was originally an aspect of women's ritual life. As he writes, 'culture begins with a tendency toward menstrual synchrony' which 'determines the symbolic language on the basis of which ritual power is expressed.' However, in certain regions or at 'certain epochs the synchrony breaks down, its formal structures are ritually preserved by men, whose tendencies toward dominance cannot now so effectively be checked' (Knight 1988: 248). Elaborating on this idea, he avers that 'the formal structures of men's rule in the Australian Aboriginal societies … bear the stamp of feminine menstrual ritual' and that 'the entire structure and language of ritual potency is derived by men from the opposite sex' (Knight 1988: 253 and 51). This derivation, in Knight's view, is one that serves the purposes of social integration and cooperation; as he writes, 'all such intimate encounters with a Snake or Rainbow or Mother, are male replications of the female potentiality to conjoin, through menstrual synchrony, in a blood-union transcending the boundaries of the self' (Knight 1988: 251).

Such blood union is evident in the initiation rites of young men. One of the intriguing aspects of such rituals is the way young boys are separated from the maternal domain of life; yet paradoxically, the symbolic nature of ritual transformation is derived from the female domain of reproduction. As noted above, male ritual represents a merging of feminine and masculine aspects of culture. For example, echoing Jung's comment on the Kundalini serpent above, among some groups, the Rainbow Snake is identified as the Mother and the ceremonial ground represents her womb. As the Berndts write, 'the ceremonial ground is symbolically identified as … the Mother.' When the men dance on the ceremonial ground, dramatising the actions of the ancestral beings of the creative period, they are 're-enacting their original spiritual conception and birth from the Mother' as well as returning to her and 'becoming sacred through entering her and being in her presence' (Berndt and Berndt 1988: 279).

On this sacred ceremonial ground, the transition of young boys into men involves them entering a symbolic representation of the uterus of the creative ancestor and being reborn as adult members of their community. For example, initiation rituals often involve the initiate being buried in a large hole dug in the ground covered with leaves, which symbolises the uterus or womb of the Fertility Mother. When the boys emerge from this symbolic uterus, they are considered to have been reborn – a rebirth that enacts the original act of primordial creation (Berndt and Berndt 1988: 252–6 and 76–87). They are then taken to where 'The Mother is said to manifest herself' during which they develop 'a lively dread that they will actually be swallowed and vomited' (Stanner 2014: 6 and 12). Significantly, Stanner argues that the 'combinations of mime, song, dance and stylised movements' during such rituals result in quite profound alterations of personality. Additionally, the symbolic forms used in such rituals primarily engage analogical thought processes that result in a deepening of the initiates 'interior life' (Stanner 2014: 26). This transformation is not one of the intellect, but emanates from what Stanner calls 'primitive intuition' (Stanner 2014: 152).

This process of transformation seems to be primarily focussed on symbolic, analogical and affect-based modes of cognition, processes that Jung argued are related to phylogenetically ancient brain systems. The appropriateness of a Jungian approach to the analysis of such ritual is further evident in Stanner's belief that it is not the ego or logical reason that is necessarily transformed, but the deeper emotional life of the initiate. As Stanner avers, the ritual evinces 'little evidence of abstract, explicit teaching' yet the 'affective outcome is most marked. Personality may almost be seen to change under one's eyes' (Stanner 2014: 22). Significantly, such a transformation results 'neural or cortical changes' (Stanner 2014: 21).

Such rites are resonant with the Iboga ceremonies discussed in Chapter 5 in which the participant is believed to regress to infancy, enter the womb and hence become more closely connected to the ancestors (Fernandez 1982: 491). They also evoke the association between the philosopher's stone and the child in its mother's womb elaborated by Jung in his study of alchemical symbolism (Jung 1983: 79–80) as well as the association between serpent imagery, maternal figures and the womb of the earth noted by both Jung and Neumann (Neumann 1954: 48–9; Jung 2014a: 200, 2014d: 436)

Jung, Ritual and Yoga

In regard to ritual, Jung argued that while psychology had revealed the biological aspect of the psyche, it had still yet to adequately explore the spiritual aspect. As he writes:

> If modern psychology can boast of having removed any of the veils which hid the psyche from us, it is only that one which had concealed from the investigator the psyche's biological aspect. We may compare the present situation to the state of medicine in the sixteenth century, when people began to study anatomy but had not as yet the faintest idea of physiology. So, too, the spiritual aspect of the psyche is known to us only in a very fragmentary way. We have learnt that there are spiritual processes of transformation in the psyche which underlie, for example, the well-known initiation rites of primitive peoples and the states induced by the practice of yoga. But we have not yet succeeded in determining their particular laws.
>
> (Jung 2014c: 462)

It is significant that in the above passage, Jung associates yoga with the rites of Indigenous or what he calls primitive peoples. This is an idea that was explored by Mircea Eliade in his *Shamanism: Archaic Techniques of Ecstasy* as well as *Yoga: Immortality and Freedom* (Eliade 1964, 2009). While Eliade noted differences between shamanism and modern yoga, he did postulate possible linkages, with shamanism evolving into a protohistocial form of yoga in which the cultivation of ecstatic states shows some affinities with yoga (Eliade 1964: 417). Significantly, Jung argued that archetypal experiences of the *numinous* 'can be traced back to their archaic roots, i.e., to ideas and images that we meet in the most ancient records and in primitive societies.' He goes on to call the reader's attention to Eliade's study of shamanism 'where a great many illuminating examples may be found' (Jung 2014b: 253).

Significantly, the association between Indigenous rituals and yoga was made by the Australian anthropologist A.P. Elkin (1891–1979) in his *Aboriginal Men of High Degree: Initiation and Sorcery in the World's Oldest Religion* several years before Eliade published *Shamanism*. Although Elkin did not use the word shaman, Eliade argued that Australian medicine men exhibited the same elements evident in global shamanism.

Elkin compiled data from across the continent on Indigenous medicine men or healers. Significantly, the book contains a section entitled 'Comparison with Tibet' where he links Australian religious practices and serpent symbolism with Kundalini yoga. For example, Elkin describes the position below the navel where the hidden abode of the sleeping Goddess Kundalini resides, the personification of the Serpent-Power or latent mystic force of the body. He compares the Goddess Kundalini and the yogic practice of cultivating internal 'psychic heat' with Australian medicine men and the imagery of the 'rainbow serpent' central to the development 'of the Australian man of high degree' (Elkin 1993: 59–60).

It is important to note that, in addition to Spencer and Gillen's *The Northern Tribes of Central Australia*, Elkin's *Aboriginal Men of High Degree* was one of the main sources on Australian initiation and medicine men that Eliade used in *Shamanism* (Eliade 1964: 45–50, 135–8 and 86). And it was Eliade's work, along with Spencer and Gillen writings on the Aranda, that was among the main sources for Jung in his writings on shamanism, crystals, sacred stones and Aboriginal religion.

In *Alchemical Studies*, as noted in Chapter 2, Jung connects the philosopher's stone or *lapis philosophicus* with cross-cultural beliefs about the sacredness of stones. In that discussion, I mentioned Jung's use of Spencer and Gillen's account in *The Northern Tribes of Central Australia* of the ritual use of *churingas* associated with the 'Alcheringa history of the snake' (Spencer and Gillen 1904: 277). In his discussion of cross-cultural stone symbolism, Jung also used Eliade's *Shamanism* as a source when connecting Australian beliefs about *churingas*, crystals and sacred stones to global motifs in shamanism. As he writes, sacred and precious stones in more recent periods probably have a very ancient pedigree and can be traced back to a 'palaeolithic cult of *churinga*-like soul-stones' (Jung 1953: 100). Jung summarises these connections providing a footnote with Eliade as his source:

> In shamanism, much importance is attached to crystals, which play the part of ministering spirits. They come from the crystal throne of the supreme being or from the vault of the sky. They show what is going on in the world and what is happening to the souls of the sick, and they also give man the power to fly.
>
> (Jung 1953: 101)

Eliade developed the connection between ancient shamanism and yoga further in his 1958 *Yoga: Immortality and Freedom* in which he wrote:

> This shamanic complex is very old; it is found, in whole or in part, among the Australians, the archaic peoples of North and South America, in the polar regions, etc. The essential and defining element of shamanism is ecstasy—the shaman is a specialist in the sacred, able to abandon his body and undertake cosmic journeys "in the spirit."
>
> (in trance) (Eliade 2009: 320)

This is a work that to my knowledge Jung never read – and it is unlikely that he would have done so as it was published near the end of his life. What seems to have been important for his theories on trance, shamanism, Indigenous cultures and yoga (what Jung called 'spiritual processes of transformation') is Eliade's earlier book where these connections are made. Additionally, Elkin had made these connections six years before Eliade published his book on shamanism.

One of the central components of the 'making' of a medicine man discussed by Elkin is his encounter with the Rainbow Snake, often in pools or rivers where he may also acquire the crystals that are essential aspects of his vocation. We can see here that medicine men are associated with imagery and symbolism taken from the maternal domain, imagery that has affinities with the serpents, water and the endogamous 'blood relations' recounted in the Wawilak Sisters Dreaming story quoted above. It is the fact that Aboriginal medicine men enter visionary states involving serpent imagery that led Elkin to make comparisons with yogic traditions. Additionally, such visionary states not only show affinities with the Wawilak Sisters Dreaming but also the initiation ceremonies discussed above in which boys are reborn from a symbolic uterus – a rebirth that enacts the original act of primordial creation (Berndt and Berndt 1988: 252–6 and 76–87). For example, one of the central components in the making of a medicine man is that, to quote Elkin, the 'postulant is swallowed by a mythical snake and reborn as a child' (Elkin 1993: 107).

Such an entry into a maternal womb like figure as a condition for rebirth and spiritual transformation is similar to the experience of regressing to infancy and life in the womb noted in Chapter 5 in the discussion of the African psychedelic Bwiti cult (Fernandez 1982: 491). The Australian example, as intimated by Elkin himself, suggests affinities with the Kundalini serpent discussed by Jung which is believed to reside in the abdominal cavity at the base of spine as well as in caves or the womb of the earth (Jung 2014d: 436).

Symbolic aspects of human culture, such as serpent and feminine imagery, as well as the child and rebirth archetype, have been long analysed by Jungians. However, there has been very little attempt to place these archetypal themes within a Darwinian framework. This may be due to the fact that evolutionary theory has tended to not study these phenomena or seek explanations for them. Knight's *Blood Relations* and consequent work building on his framework have changed that situation offering a Darwinian account of many of the motifs discussed in this study

(Knight 1995; Finnegan 2013; Power, Finnegan, and Callan 2017). There are deep affinities between the paradigm developed by Knight and colleagues and the material analysed by Jungians. This may be because Knight was in part inspired by *The Wise Wound: Menstruation and Everywoman* by Peter Redgrove and Penelope Shuttle, a Jungian analysis of menstruation and its importance to human cultural life (Shuttle and Redgrove 1978; Knight 1995: 37).

In this study, I have sought to bring Knight's evolutionary model and analytical psychology into dialogue. This approach I believe can be extremely generative in grounding archetypal psychology in evolutionary theory. However, I have only really been able to touch the surface of what is a rich subject that warrants much deeper and extensive investigation. It is my hope that other researchers will investigate the issues I have raised in this study and explore further the affinities between the evolutionary paradigm developed by Knight and colleagues and analytical psychology.

References

Bell, D. 2002. *Daughters of the Dreaming* (Spinifex Press).

Bell, D., and T.N. Nelson. 1989. 'Speaking about Rape Is Everyone's Business', *Women's Studies International Forum*, 12: 403–16.

Berndt, R.M., and C.H. Berndt. 1951. *Sexual Behavior in Western Arnhem Land* (University of California).

Berndt, R.M., and C.H. Berndt. 1988. *The World of the First Australians: Aboriginal Traditional Life: Past and Present* (Aboriginal Studies Press).

Bulkeley, K. 2016. *Big Dreams: The Science of Dreaming and the Origins of Religion* (Oxford University Press).

Carhart-Harris, R.L., and K.J. Friston. 2019. 'REBUS and the Anarchic Brain: Toward a Unified Model of the Brain Action of Psychedelics', *Pharmacological Reviews*, 71: 316.

Carhart-Harris, R.L., R. Leech, P.J. Hellyer, M. Shanahan, A. Feilding, E. Tagliazucchi, et al. 2014. 'The Entropic Brain: A Theory of Conscious States Informed by Neuroimaging Research with Psychedelic Drugs', *Frontiers in Human Neuroscience*, 8: 149–64.

Clark, G. 2014. 'Speaking Out on Aboriginal Violence', *Quadrant*, 58: 69–73.

Clark, G., C. Barlow, V. Polito, and A. Wilkes. 2017. Barlow, C. Polito, V. Wilkes, A. 'The Dionysian Primate: The Default Mode Network, Psychopathology and the Psychedelic Brain.' In *Entheogenesis Australis Psychedelic Symposium 2017*, 25–27 (Entheogenesis Australis).

Clark, G. 2022. 'Review of the Path of the Serpent, Volume 1: Psychedelics and the Neuropsychology of Gnosis by Hereward Tilton', *Journal of Jungian Scholarly Studies*, 17: 95–8.

Daws, R., C. Timmermann, B. Giribaldi, J. Sexton, M. Wall, D. Erritzoe, et al. 2022. 'Increased Global Integration in the Brain after Psilocybin Therapy for Depression', *Nature Medicine*, 28: 844–51.

Dunbar, R. 2014. *Human Evolution: A Pelican Introduction* (Penguin Books Limited).

Dussart, F. 2000. *The Politics of Ritual in an Aboriginal Settlement: Kinship, Gender, and the Currency of Knowledge* (Smithsonian Institution Press).

Eliade, M. 1964. *Shamanism: Archaic Techniques of Ecstasy* (Bollingen Foundation).

Eliade, M. 2009. *Yoga: Immortality and Freedom* (Princeton University Press).

Elkin, A.P. 1993. *Aboriginal Men of High Degree: Initiation and Sorcery in the World's Oldest Tradition* (Inner Traditions/Bear).

Fernandez, J.W. 1982. *Bwiti: An Ethnography of the Religious Imagination in Africa* (Princeton University Press).

Finnegan, M. 2013. 'The Politics of Eros: Ritual Dialogue and Egalitarianism in Three Central African Hunter-Gatherer Societies', *Journal of the Royal Anthropological Institute*, 19: 697–715.

Flor-Henry, P., Y. Shapiro, C. Sombrun, and P. Walla. 2017. 'Brain Changes during a Shamanic Trance: Altered Modes of Consciousness, Hemispheric Laterality, and Systemic Psychobiology', *Cogent Psychology*, 4: 1313522.

Harding, M.E. 1936. *Woman's Mysteries: Ancient and Modern* (Longman).

Hume, L. 2002. *Ancestral Power: The Dreaming, Consciousness and Aboriginal Australians* (Melbourne University Press).

James, D., E. Tregenza, A. Tjilari, K. Kankapankatja, T. Edwards, D. Miller, et al. 2014. *Ngintaka* (Wakefield Press).

Jung, C.G. 1953. *Collected Works of C. G. Jung, Volume 13: Alchemical Studies* (Princeton University Press).

Jung, C.G. 1980. *Collected Works of C.G. Jung, Volume 12: Psychology and Alchemy* (Princeton University Press).

Jung, C.G. 1983. *The Psychology of the Transference* (Routledge).

Jung, C.G. 2014a. *Collected Works of C.G. Jung, Volume 9 (Part 1): Archetypes and the Collective Unconscious* (Princeton University Press).

Jung, C.G. 2014b. *Collected Works of C.G. Jung, Volume 18: The Symbolic Life: Miscellaneous Writings* (Princeton University Press).

Jung, C.G. 2014c. *The Structure and Dynamics of the Psyche* (Taylor & Francis).

Jung, C.G. 2014d. *Symbols of Transformation* (Taylor & Francis).

Katz, R. 1982. *Boiling Energy: Community Healing among the Kalahari Kung* (Harvard University Press).

Keeney, B. 2000. *Kalahari Bushman Healers* (Leete's Island Books).

Keeney, B., and H. Keeney. 2013. 'Reentry into First Creation', *Journal of Anthropological Research*, 69: 65–86.

Kimm, J. 2004. *A Fatal Conjunction: Two Laws, Two Cultures* (Federation Press).

Knight, C. 1988. 'Menstrual Synchrony and the Australian Rainbow Snake.' in Buckley, T., and A. Gottlieb (eds.), *Blood Magic: The Anthropology of Menstruation* (University of California Press).

Knight, C. 1995. *Blood Relations: Menstruation and the Origins of Culture* (Yale University Press).

Konner, M. 2015. *Women after All: Sex, Evolution, and the End of Male Supremacy* (W. W. Norton).

Lee, R.B. 1979. *The !Kung San: Men, Women and Work in a Foraging Society* (Cambridge University Press).

Lincoln, J.S. 1970. *The Dream in Primitive Cultures* (Johnson Reprint Corporation).

Luppi, A., R. Carhart-Harris, L. Roseman, I. Pappas, D. Menon, and E. Stamatakis. 2021. 'LSD Alters Dynamic Integration and Segregation in the Human Brain', *NeuroImage*, 227: 117653.

Marshack, A. 1985. 'On the Dangers of Serpents in the Mind', *Current Anthropology*, 26: 139–52.

McNamara, P., and K. Bulkeley. 2015. 'Dreams as a Source of Supernatural Agent Concepts', *Frontiers in Psychology*, 6: 1–8.

Meggitt, M.J. 1962. *Desert People: A Study of the Walbiri Aborigines of Central Australia* (University of Chicago Press).

Munn, N.D. 1973. *Walbiri Iconography: Graphic Representation and Cultural Symbolism in a Central Australian Society* (Cornell University Press).

Neumann, E. 1954. *The Origins and History of Consciousness* (Pantheon Books).

Neumann, E. 1994. *The Fear of the Feminine: And Other Essays on Feminine Psychology* (Princeton University Press).

Perera, S.B. 1981. *Descent to the Goddess: A Way of Initiation for Women* (Inner City Books).

Pokorny, T., K.H. Preller, M. Kometer, I. Dziobek, and F.X. Vollenweider. 2017. 'Effect of Psilocybin on Empathy and Moral Decision-Making', *International Journal of Neuropsychopharmacology*, 20: 747–57.

Power, C. 2017. 'Reconstructing a Source Cosmology for African Hunter-Gatherers.' in Power, C., M. Finnegan, and H. Calla (eds.), *Human Origins: Contributions from Social Anthropology* (Berghahn Books).

Power, C. 2022. 'Lunarchy: The Original Human Economics of Time.' in Silva, F., and L. Henty (eds.), *Solarizing the Moon: Essays in Honour of Lionel Sims* (Archaeopress).

Power, C., M. Finnegan, and H. Callan. 2017. *Human Origins: Contributions from Social Anthropology* (Berghahn Books).

Preller, K., T. Pokorny, A. Hock, R. Kraehenmann, P. Stämpfli, E. Seifritz, et al. 2016. 'Effects of Serotonin 2A/1A Receptor Stimulation on Social Exclusion Processing', *Proceedings of the National Academy of Sciences*, 113: 5119–24.

Shostak, M. 2009. *Nisa: The Life and Words of a !Kung Woman* (Harvard University Press).

Shuttle, P., and P. Redgrove. 1978. *The Wise Wound: Eve's Curse and Everywoman* (Richard Marek Publishers).

Spencer, B., and F.J. Gillen. 1904. *The Northern Tribes of Central Australia* (Macmillan and Company Limited).

Spreng, R.N., R.A. Mar, and A.S.N. Kim. 2008. 'The Common Neural Basis of Autobiographical Memory, Prospection, Navigation, Theory of Mind, and the Default Mode: A Quantitative Meta-Analysis', *Journal of Cognitive Neuroscience*, 21: 489–510.

Stanner, W.E.H. 1998. 'Some Aspects of Aboriginal Religion.' in Charlesworth M. J. (ed.), *Religious Business: Essays on Australian Aboriginal Spirituality* (Cambridge University Press).

Stanner, W.E.H. 2014. *On Aboriginal Religion* (Sydney University Press).

Sutton, P. 2005. 'Rage, Reason and the Honourable Cause: A Reply to Cowlishaw', *Australian Aboriginal Studies*, 2: 35–43.

Tilton, H. 2020. *The Path of the Serpent: Psychedelics and the Neuropsychology of Gnosis, Volume 1* (Rubedo Press).

Warner, W.L. 1969. *A Black Civilization: A Social Study of an Australian Tribe* (P. Smith).

Watts, I. 2017. 'Rain Serpents in Northern Australia and Southern Africa: A Common Ancestry?' in Power, C., M. Finnegan, and H. Callan (eds.), *Human Origins* (Berghahn Books).

Winkelman, M., and M. Dobkin de Rios. 1989. 'Psychoactive Properties of !Kung Bushmen Medicine Plants', *Journal of Psychoactive Drugs*, 21: 51–9.

Zhou, H., X. Chen, Y. Shen, L. Li, N. Chen, Z. Zhu, et al. 2020. 'Rumination and the Default Mode Network: Meta-Analysis of Brain Imaging Studies and Implications for Depression', *NeuroImage*, 206: 116287.

Conclusion

Conclusion

One of the dilemmas of humans researching the evolutionary origins of consciousness is that we must use consciousness to do so. This produces a particularly difficult problem – one that Jung was acutely aware of when he wrote that he 'who would fathom the psyche must not confuse it with consciousness, else he veils from his own sight the object he wishes to explore. On the contrary, to recognise the psyche, even, he must learn to see how it differs from consciousness' (Jung 2001: 74). If consciousness, and the recently evolved brain systems that subserve it, is segregated or dissociated from phylogenetically ancient brain systems, then that recently evolved system is going to lack actual perceptual data regarding that more ancient system. This lack of perceptual data is inherent in Jung's theory of the collective unconscious – because it is unconscious, we lack conscious awareness of it.

This is a problem of profound seriousness for our culture and its political and scientific institutions as well as our therapeutic professions. It represents an inherent impasse the human mind faces in attempting to understand its own evolution and the ontogenetic and phylogenetic foundations out of which it emerged. It was this inability of consciousness to adequately research its own evolutionary foundations that Robin Carhart-Harris was referring to when he wrote that 'mainstream psychology and psychiatry have underappreciated the depth of the human mind by neglecting schools of thought that posit the existence of an unconscious mind' (Carhart-Harris et al. 2014: 18).

From the perspective of the model outlined in this book, such underappreciation is to a large extent understandable – one might even say inevitable. Scientific researchers, being members of the species *Homo sapiens*, are not immune to the dissociation or brain segregation that seems to be an evolved and inherent feature of our species-typical neural architecture. Consequently, that dissociation has informed our models of the mind and its evolution. Jung sought to address this dilemma throughout his works. He also noted that while consciousness generally lacks access to phylogenetically ancient brain systems, there are certain phenomena such as dreams and ritually induced states of

DOI: 10.4324/9781032624549-8

consciousness that permeate the barrier separating archaic from more recently evolved brain systems.

This dissociation of consciousness from its evolutionary foundations is one of the most ubiquitous features of human civilisation, although due to the nature of such dissociation, this is rarely acknowledged in accounts of human historical development. For example, accompanying such dissociation is the frequent lack of awareness that it exists. In this sense, we can become dissociated from our dissociation. This presents a problem for those researching human cultural history as some of the most important aspects of human cultural development are only explicable if we adopt an evolutionary conception of mind of the kind Jung developed. Without such a conception, much of human culture remains inexplicable – from prehistoric shamanism and the Eleusinian Mysteries, to the works of Plotinus and the Gnostics to modern writers such as Goethe.

In *The Divided Self*, R.D. Laing analysed this process of repression:

Our civilization represses not only 'the instincts', not only sexuality, but any form of transcendence … Thus I would wish to emphasize that our 'normal' 'adjusted' state is too often the abdication of ecstasy, the betrayal of our true potentialities.

(Laing 1988: 11–12)

The model outlined in this book provides an account of such abdication as an emergent phenomenon associated with the evolution and development of consciousness. It was a process that Jung traced from prehistory, through antiquity and the Middle Ages to the modern world. The virtue of Jung's approach resides in his ability to see the problem from a meta-perspective so to speak, as opposed to remaining mired in it. In this sense, he could analyse the historical trajectory of individual and collective dissociation and envision a future historical stage in which that dissociation is made an object of scientific enquiry and through that process of investigation potentially resolved. In this sense, individuation, that is, the integration of ego consciousness with the collective unconscious, is not only a personal endeavour but a historical and cultural one.

The next stage of human consciousness, from this perspective, involves emerging out of the period of Enlightenment and rationalist modernity, and into a new paradigm where dissociation from the collective unconscious is a phenomenon humans become increasingly aware of. And through that process of conscious awareness begin to heal the split inherent within the evolved structure of the human brain itself. For while phylogenetic dispositions can be negated, forgotten or dissociated through individual, cultural or historical processes, this does not mean that such dispositions are irretrievably lost as the quest for understating them can lead to holistic integration (Mills 2010; Clark 2022: 325).

Jung was limited in the degree he could achieve such integration due to the state of science during the time he lived. Nevertheless, he pointed the way towards what such a paradigm may look like. With the development of modern neuroimaging techniques, and the growth in psychedelic neuroscience, the ability of our species to probe the heretofore hidden depths of the human mind has reached a new level of sophistication Jung could not have imagined.

From early hominins such as *Ardipithecus ramidus*, with their ape-like cognitive ontogeny, to *Homo erectus* with its extended life history, all the way through to the scientific revolution and the present, human consciousness has been evolving. Jung's work was an important advance in that evolutionary and historical development of consciousness. Today however, we can build on and extend his insights and deepen and refine our empirical grasp of the human mind, how it evolved and what is the relationship between our minds and those of the diverse range of species we share the planet with. In this sense, we are entering a new stage of consciousness beyond that envisioned by Jung. However, his voluminous works provide a compass and a system of orientation that can inform and enrich our understanding of the nature of consciousness and its archaic evolutionary foundations. Those works will no doubt also inform the developing science of consciousness and our species' growing self-awareness of its origins. As we head into an uncertain future, such self-awareness will be crucial if our species is to flourish and avoid civilisational and planetary collapse.

References

Carhart-Harris, R.L., R. Leech, P.J. Hellyer, M. Shanahan, A. Feilding, E. Tagliazucchi, et al. 2014. 'The Entropic Brain: A Theory of Conscious States Informed by Neuroimaging Research with Psychedelic Drugs', *Frontiers in Human Neuroscience*, 8: 149–64.
Clark, G. 2022. 'The Dionysian Primate: Goethe, Nietzsche, Jung and Psychedelic Neuroscience.' in Miils J., and D. Burston (eds.), *Psychoanalysis and the Mind-Body Problem* (Rouledge).
Jung, C.G. 2001. *Modern Man in Search of a Soul* (Routledge).
Laing, R.D. 1988. *The Divided Self: An Existential Study in Sanity and Madness* (Penguin Books).
Mills, J. 2010. *Origins: On the Genesis of Psychic Reality* (McGill-Queen's University Press).

Index

For Product Safety Concerns and Information please contact our EU
representative GPSR@taylorandfrancis.com
Taylor & Francis Verlag GmbH, Kaufingerstraße 24, 80331 München, Germany

9 781032 624518